Your Brain and Nerves

J. Lawrence Pool, M. D.

Your Brain
and
Nerves

CHARLES SCRIBNER'S SONS

NEW YORK

To my wife, Angeline

Contents

Preface

A neurosurgeon, in order to operate on the brain, spinal cord, and nerves, must—during the course of five to seven years of training after medical school—learn many details concerning the structure, electricity, and chemistry of the nervous system. For a neurosurgeon is the specialist who is called upon to remove brain tumors and slipped discs, to repair injured nerves, or to remedy, when possible, certain inborn, or congenital, defects that cripple children and certain kinds of strokes that afflict older persons. But to do these things he must have much more than a pair of skilled hands. To use his skills in the ancient art of healing the sick, he must also have a working knowledge of the research that has been done and is being done on the nervous system and the various organs associated with it. And he must understand how the circulation of blood and the flow of the cerebrospinal fluid in the head can go wrong and be remedied in order to treat dangerous conditions they may cause. He needs an awareness of all the chemical agents that can relieve pain, epilepsy, brain congestion, and defective circulation of the blood, and must be familiar with means of helping nerves regrow and muscles recover after serious injuries.

In addition to this, a conscientious neurosurgeon does his best to offer his patients and their families a generous measure of human understanding, helping them, whenever possible, to overcome their fears, and supplanting needless worries with reassuring explanations. He relieves the anxious mother of a child with a skull fracture by explaining that the fracture itself is often harmless provided the brain has not been seriously injured. He explains to patients the purpose of a spinal tap and, when the occasion demands, makes sure that the patient and members of his family have the facts on which to base an informed choice as to whether or not an operation or some other kind of treatment is advisable. He promises no miracles, but explains what could happen if indicated surgery were not performed. It is my earnest hope that the explanations in this book will reduce the natural apprehension that people have regarding the clearly remediable conditions with which neurosurgeons deal.

It is in this same spirit that I have written this book. The book is, in part, an attempt to reach out to those who are in need of information and to set on paper some of the exchanges that have taken place with my patients. It is also an attempt to set forth some of the tremendous strides taken in research during the past few years. The amount that has been learned during my own professional lifetime alone is astounding, taking in everything from surgery for mental illnesses and pain to the prevention and alleviation of certain previously untreatable strokes, brain tumors, and acute spinal injuries.

The numerous case histories in this book are not actual individual cases. Some are combinations of various aspects of many real cases. In others, circumstances have been slightly altered to fit better into the context of the story. Still others are fictional variations of similar incidents which actually occurred. For the privacy of the patients from whose experiences I have drawn, the individuals in the histories are referred to by fictional initials.

Grateful acknowledgment is made to Patricia Lauber for her expert editorial assistance and to my neurosurgical colleagues at the Neurological Institute of New York, Columbia-Presbyterian Medical Center, for their kindness in supplying helpful suggestions for this book. I also wish to thank Dr. C. Paul O'Connell for reviewing the completed text.

Your Brain and Nerves

Introduction

Everything we know about the world about us comes to us through our senses—through our nerves. And every different kind of sensation, whether it is smell, vision, pain, or touch, is detected by a different kind of nerve cell whose job it is to sense that particular kind of sensation, and, generally speaking, no other. This means that nature has provided one set of sensing cells for vision, for example, and another variety for pain. Once detected by the sensing, or sensory, cells of the body, sensations are flashed to the spinal cord or directly to the brain itself by signals that speed along nerves at rates of up to 200 miles an hour. When these signals reach the spinal cord or brain, they are immediately modulated as to intensity —as if by the volume control of a radio set—and also promptly sorted out for relay to appropriate parts of the cord or brain. The modulation, sorting, and relaying is performed by clusters of nerve cells inside the cord and brain. Each of these cell clusters therefore acts like a miniature computer which interprets incoming messages and then decides, within a split second, whether or not to send other messages back to body structures such as the muscles and glands to tell them what or what not to do. In simple terms, this means that our daily activities, including our conscious life, depend on our nervous system: our nerves, spinal cord, and brain.

Of these three components of the nervous system, the brain is paramount. It is also one of the most extraordinary structures on earth, beside which man's most sophisticated computers pale into insignificance. This is because of the brain's marvelous compactness, magnificent efficiency, and wide range of potential responses. These responses, whether they are complex thoughts, expressions of emotion, or coordinated muscle action, are all mediated by millions upon millions of tiny nerve cells, visible only with a microscope, that are packed closely together in various parts of the spinal cord and the brain. Their small size and dense packaging accounts for the compactness of the brain and cord.

The efficiency of the brain and cord is accounted for by other factors. One of these is the automatically regulated fuel system—the circulation of blood—which is the source of nourishment for nerve cells. The circulating blood also helps maintain an even temperature and a favorable balance of the chemical substances necessary for their efficient performance. Another factor is the natural liquid, as crystal clear as spring water, which, from the moment life begins, bathes the entire brain and spinal cord. This liquid, called the cerebrospinal fluid, shares with the circulating blood the role of maintaining a favorable chemical climate for the brain and cord and assists in carrying away waste products of their metabolism. A third factor is the ability of each tiny nerve cell to generate its own electrical power and to manufacture the chemicals necessary for the transmission of nerve signals. This means that every nerve cell, whether it is in the body—as the sensory cells are—or actually inside the brain or cord, is at the same time both a miniature electrical power plant and a chemical factory. For every nerve signal depends on an electrical charge generated in a nerve cell, and on special chemical substances called neuro- (nerve) transmitter substances made by a nerve cell. Some of these transmitter substances are also manufactured by the filamentous, whiskerlike extensions of nerve cells called nerve fibers.

To look at the brain one would scarcely dream that it is such a marvelous electrical and chemical apparatus. Roughly melon-shaped, it looks and feels like a mass of grayish-white, rather solid jelly. Its surface has a somewhat crumpled appearance caused by its folds, called convolutions, which are separated from each other by thin clefts, or fissures, about half an inch in depth. The largest or uppermost part of the brain is divided from front to back into two halves known as the cerebral hemispheres. Under them, at the extreme back of the head, there is another portion, smaller in size and a little different in appearance, called the cerebellum or "little brain." And under this, at the very base of the brain, there is a column of brain tissue—the stem of the brain, or brainstem—which connects the brain with the spinal cord.

In popular parlance the part of the brain that does the thinking is generally spoken of as the "gray matter." Actually there is a lot of gray matter that does much more than this. Some of it, for example, is principally concerned with the receipt and interpretation of messages from the outside world and from the body itself. Another section is largely responsible for sending nerve signals back to the body, while still other portions deal mainly with the storage and recall of memories or with the control of our emotions.

The term gray matter is derived from the fact that

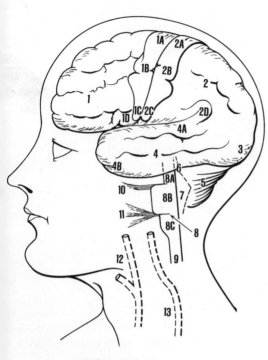

1 frontal lobe
  1A leg area of motor strip
  1B hand area of motor strip
  1C face area of motor strip
  1D a speech-control area
2 parietal lobe
  2A leg area of sensory strip
  2B hand area of sensory strip
  2C face area of sensory strip
  2D a major speech-control area
3 occipital lobe concerned with vision
4 temporal lobe
  4A hearing area of cortex
  4B area involved in psychomotor epilepsy
5 cerebellum, concerned with balance and coordination
6 aqueduct of Sylvius, for escape of CSF
7 fourth ventricle
8 brainstem
  8A midbrain
  8B pons (nerve "bridge")
  8C medulla
9 spinal cord
10 cranial nerve III (eye movements)
11 cranial nerve V (facial sensations and chewing)
12 carotid artery
13 vertebral artery

BRAIN: *Above:* side view;
below: cross section

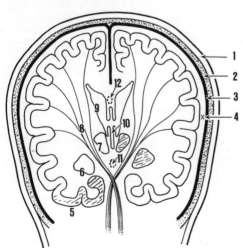

1 scalp
2 skull bone (*stippled*)
3 dura (*heavy black line*)
4 space filled with CSF
5 cortex (gray matter)
6 basal ganglia (deep gray matter)
7 thalamus (deep gray matter)
8 nerve fibers (crossing in the brainstem)
9 lateral ventricle
10 third ventricle
11 pituitary gland (*dotted circle*)
12 pineal gland (*dotted circle*)

SPINAL CORD AND NERVES
Above: side view;
below: cross section. Numbers
on both refer to the legend.

1 vertebral body
2 opening for nerve
3 joint
4 lamina
5 spinous process
6 dura (*heavy black line*)
7 spinal cord (*gray matter stippled*)
8 sensory nerve root
9 motor nerve root
10 nerve formed by a sensory and
    a motor root
11 autonomic ("automatic") nerve
    chain
12 nerve pathway of spinal cord
13 disc (note proximity to nerves)

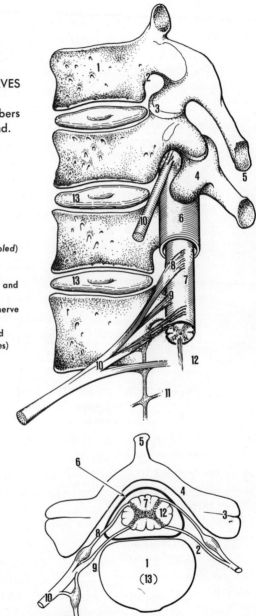

certain portions of the brain and spinal cord have a grayish color wherever there are either dense layers or dense clusters of nerve cells. This explains why the entire surface of the cerebral hemispheres and the cerebellum has a grayish hue. For the brain's surface consists principally of a layer of closely packed nerve cells. Despite the thinness of this layer—only about an eighth of an inch—the harmonious action and interaction of all its cells make possible such activities as constructive thinking, the appreciation of art, and the ability to hit a home run or play a violin.

Immediately under the surface gray matter lies the white matter, which is white because it contains no nerve cells and is composed mainly of nerve fibers, which, unlike nerve cells, are pale rather than gray. Sandwiched deep down in the brain's white matter, however, there are several large clusters of nerve cells which, like the surface nerve cells, impart a gray color to these clusters. These deep cell groups, which modulate and relay nerve messages, are referred to as the deep gray matter.

The spinal cord—really an extension of the brain—also contains both gray and white matter. Running up and down its entire core, for example, there are large numbers of nerve cells that make this innermost portion of the cord look gray. All messages between the brain and the body are relayed through these cells. They also make possible reflexes, such as the jerk of your leg when a doctor taps your knee, by locally relaying incoming nerve signals directly back to the leg muscles. All around the central core of gray matter lie closely packed nerve fibers—the white matter of the cord—which transmit all messages between the cord and the brain in both an upward and a downward direction.

Another miracle of the nervous system is how small a structure the spinal cord is, compared to what it does for us. Without it we could not, for example, sit up, stand, walk, or even feed ourselves. We could not even tell whether our hands and feet were hot or cold. Yet this main nerve cable of the body is no bigger around than the diameter of one's index finger. It runs all the way from the back of the head to the level of the lowest or twelfth rib, well protected within a tubelike canal of bone formed by the spinal bones or vertebrae. Below the twelfth rib the bony spinal canal is filled with branches of the nerves that supply the legs, bladder, and lower bowel.

The wiring system of the body itself consists of its nerves. They are all connected either to the spinal cord or the brain. Those of the head, because they are connected directly with the brain, are called cranial nerves. There are twelve on each side: the first, or farthest forward, being the nerve for the sense of smell—the olfactory nerve—while the last or farthest back, the twelfth, is the one which makes the tongue muscles move. The nerves of the body, which are called peripheral nerves, are made up, just outside the spinal bones, by the union of small nerve branches called nerve roots, which emerge from the spinal cord. From head to tail, on each side of the spine, there are thirty of these nerve roots, each of which leaves the spinal canal through a small opening between two adjacent vertebrae.

A nerve—which is essentially a cable, rather than a wire—whether it is short or long, small or large in diameter, is a round, glistening white, flexible structure having a rubbery consistency. The longest and largest is the sciatic nerve. At its uppermost portion it is roughly as big around as one's index finger but becomes smaller by tapering out as various branches leave it on their way to muscles or the skin of the leg, on its long course from the spine all the way down to the toes.

These and many other details concerning nerves, spinal cord, and brain are part of the basic information which the neurosurgeon applies to the diagnosis and treatment of disease and injury to these components of our vastly complex and efficient nervous system.

1

The
Aching Back

Disc Damage

Of all the ailments that may afflict the human spine, a damaged disc is one of the most common. It usually leads to a low-back or leg pain that may clear up after a few days or plague a person on and off for years. In rare cases it may cause such instant and enduring pain that prompt admission to a hospital is required.

Various thoughts occur to people when a disc first causes trouble. Many, and probably most, people think, "I've sprained a muscle in my back." And this is, in fact, by far the most common cause of an aching back. A few may say to themselves, "If it's a disc, maybe I'll be paralyzed, or—dare I think it—maybe it's cancer." Such worries should really be laid to rest. Discs very, very rarely lead to any paralysis, and even if they do, it can be corrected by prompt treatment. Cancer, or even a benign tumor, is the least likely cause of an aching back.

Disc trouble can happen to anyone, regardless of age, sex, or occupation, and the damage can be incurred in a number of ways. It can occur, for example, simply as a result of wear and tear on a disc and its binding ligaments in persons unusually susceptible to disc disease. It can also occur as the result of a long-past or recent strain or injury, as illustrated by the cases of three fairly typical patients.

Mr. N., an office worker unused to heavy physical labor, pitched in to help a moving man. He lifted a large box of books by bending at the waist, seizing the box, and then straightening up. Doing so, he felt, as he later said, "something happen in my back." The next morning he became aware of such pain and stiffness in the small of the back (lumbago) that he could not straighten up while shaving. Gradually the painful stiffness subsided sufficiently so that he managed his usual trip to the office. But all that day and for the next three days he experienced much the same discomfort. By the end of a week, however, he felt fine.

Two years later, while standing by his desk, he turned quickly to pick up some papers. Immediately a pain so sharp that it almost made him fall shot all the way down his left leg from hip to toes. This pain, sciatica, was so severe that he had to lie down. The company physician gave him "pain pills" and arranged for him to be driven home for rest in bed and treatment by his own doctor.

Miss L., an active young woman in good physical trim, twisted her body in a desperate effort to make a difficult return on the tennis court and felt a sudden pain in the lower part of her back that coursed immediately down the back of the right leg. She crumpled to the ground and later that day had to be taken to the local hospital because the pain was so severe.

Mr. W. was driving a pickup truck when he was involved in a rear-end collision that snapped his head back, leaving him with pain in the back of the neck and also pain, tingling, and numbness down the right arm to the thumb, index, and middle fingers. When these symptoms failed to improve, his doctor, calling it a whiplash injury, insisted on prompt admission to a hospital for x-rays and other appropriate tests and treatment.

All three persons, as it turned out, had damaged a disc, one of the cushions of cartilage that separate the vertebrae, causing it to bulge or rupture (a "slipped disc"). The pain that each person immediately or subsequently felt was caused by the disc's pressing on, or "pinching," a nerve root inside the spine.

Except in extreme cases, a diagnosis of disc disease may take time to arrive at, for the symptoms it induces can equally well have a number of other causes. So that a patient may understand this and also the nature of his problem, I find it helpful in talking with him to begin at the beginning, by explaining the spine itself.

The Structure of the Spine

The human spine is a remarkable structure. It is strong enough to support most of the body's weight, yet flexible enough so that a person can bend down to touch his toes. In addition, it is the sole protection for the spinal cord and for all the nerve roots of the cord that join together outside the spine to form the nerves of the body.

Body support is provided by the vertebrae, a series of bones that rest one on top of another, like a column of children's blocks. The column is flexible because the vertebrae are linked by joints that lock them together and yet permit some degree of motion. Each vertebra is separated from its neighbor by a disc, which is a circular piece of cartilage, or gristle, one-eighth to one-fourth inch thick, with something of the consistency of a large, tough clam.

The discs act as cushions that not only separate adjacent vertebrae but, by their rubbery resiliency, contribute to the flexibility of the spine. Each disc is held in place and contained by a thick ringlike ligament of its own and also by ligaments of the spine. If there were no discs, the spinal bones would be in direct contact with one another and would either grind together or make the spine as stiff and inflexible as a poker.

In all, there are twenty-four jointed vertebrae: seven in the neck, twelve corresponding to the twelve ribs, and five forming the lower part of the spine known as the lumbar region or "small of the back."

The spine ends on the sacrum, a solid wedge of bone formed of five solidly fused vertebrae that resemble one solid piece of bone. The sacrum, like the keystone of an arch, fits firmly between the two iliac, or hip, bones and locks them together at the sacroiliac joints. (The latter, however, are seldom the cause of pain despite the popular beliefs to this effect some years ago.)

The spine tapers off in the coccyx, or tail-bone, which consists of three very small fused vertebrae. The tails of dogs and other animals contain several of these terminal vertebrae, but obviously they are not fused in animals that wag their tails!

The blocklike body of every vertebra has a backward extension on each side. These join to form an arch of bone. The right and the left segments of this arch are wing-shaped and each is called a lamina.

Each arch, from its apex or farthest back portion, gives rise to a spike of bone called the spinous process. The rounded tips of these spikes are the bumps one can see and feel under the skin all along the middle of one's back. They are useful landmarks for doctors preparing to do a spinal tap and for surgeons who operate on the spine.

Between the body of each vertebra and its laminal arch there is a hollow ring-shaped space. Together all the ring-shaped spaces up and down the spine form a canal called the spinal canal. The canal contains the spinal cord and its nerve branches called nerve roots. The canal is essentially a flexible tube of bone with the diameter of a large garden hose. It is lined throughout by ligaments that help hold the vertebral bones together and also serve as a protective covering for the spinal cord. Just inside the ligaments lining the spinal canal there is a layer of soft fat and then a thick bluish membrane, the dura, both of which surround the spinal cord. Immediately beneath this dural inner tube there is cerebrospinal fluid, usually referred to as CSF, contained by two very thin transparent inner membranes. The spinal cord lies within this water jacket and is therefore very well protected, having, like a series of Chinese boxes, six coverings: the skin and muscles, the spinal bones, their binding inner ligaments, an encircling cushion of fat, a tube of dura, and finally a water jacket.

The spinal cord is the cable that connects the brain with the body. It is a white flexible oval structure continuous with the medulla or lowermost part of the brain. Before birth the spinal cord extends all the way down to the sacrum, but as the spine grows, the cord is pulled upward until in adults its lower end is at the level of the twelfth rib. From this level down to the sacrum, the spinal canal is filled with the nerve roots of the spinal cord. These lower roots, closely packed together, look like the hairs of a horse's tail and have therefore been called the cauda equina, from the Latin *cauda* (tail) and *equina* (horse).

The nerve roots of the spinal cord are delicate glistening white strands composed of many fine nerve fibers that enter and leave both sides of the spinal cord through bony openings between the vertebrae. Immediately outside the spine the nerve roots join together to form the nerves of the body.

If a nerve root is compressed, pain is an almost certain consequence. There may also be numbness in the part of the body supplied by sensation-carrying fibers of the nerve root. Pressure on the nerve fibers in the roots that activate muscles may cause weakness and eventually withering of the muscles they supply.

Compression of a nerve root can have various causes, among them a disc that is bulging or one that has actually ruptured through its containing ligaments, much as a caterpillar ruptures when stepped on. Either a bulging or a ruptured disc can lead to the same symptoms.

When Mr. N., the office worker, lifted the heavy box of books, he put so much strain on one disc in his lower back that it was partly crushed. It thus became softened instead of being firm and rubbery. At the same time the ligaments holding it in place became stretched and so weakened by the unaccustomed strain that the softened disc material tended to bulge into the spinal canal. Here the disc pressed on a nerve root, causing a reflex spasm of the back muscles that led to the pain and stiffness he experienced. (Since a disc itself has no nerves, it is not the source of the pain it may induce. However, the spine's ligaments just inside the disc do have nerves, that can lead to local backache when the ligaments are stretched by a bulging disc.)

With the passage of time and the avoidance of further strain, pain from a bulging disc very often goes away, as it did initially in the case of Mr. N. This is either because the bulging part of the disc returns to its normal position so that it no longer presses on a nerve or ligament, or because the nerve root adapts to mild pressure from a disc. Many people never have any further trouble after an initial episode, presumably because the healing process of the weakened ligaments keeps the disc placed where it belongs. In some less fortunate individuals, however, like Mr. N., the containing ligaments may gradually become weaker rather than stronger with time, and the disc progressively softer, or more "degenerated," until very little is required to cause it to burst its bonds and rupture, or herniate. This is what happened two years later when Mr. N. turned quickly to pick up his papers. The turning tended to split apart the strands of weak ligament and allow the underlying disc to rupture and thus press upon the nerve root over it. "I think the time has now come," said his doctor, "for you to see a specialist." Mr. N. agreed.

In the second case, Miss L. obviously suffered an immediate disc rupture as the result of her lunge on the tennis court. Her back strain was such that the internal spinal ligaments immediately gave way and the disc popped out, although there had been no previous back trouble.

As Mr. W.'s case shows, discs may cause trouble in the neck as well as in the lower back. These two regions, the mid-portion of the neck and the lowermost part of the lumbar spine, are most commonly afflicted because they are the most mobile parts of the spine and therefore subject to more wear, tear, and strain than those elsewhere. The sudden snap of the head and neck sustained by Mr. W., for example, so abruptly and powerfully compressed a neck disc that it popped out like a pea from a pod. Like lower discs, however, neck discs sometimes return to their normal position with relief of symptoms, while in other cases, like Mr. W.'s, they may remain in a ruptured position and cause continued pain and other symptoms. Fortunately, most whiplash injuries of the neck do not result in disc damage.

Diagnosis and Treatment

What should people do when these kinds of back or neck pain and other symptoms occur? I feel it is best for them to consult their own physician promptly so that he can evaluate the situation and advise treatment. Self-care may mean that the person does not rest when he should, or returns to commuting or to work at a time when jostling on a train, bus, or elevator either slows recovery or precipitates new symptoms. Another reason for prompt medical evaluation is to obtain a record of symptoms, reflex activity, and other details as a basis for comparison with any possible future developments. It is also important to obtain x-rays to rule out a fracture.

Should pain or any other symptoms fail to improve, become worse, or be severe and crippling from the start, a specialist should be consulted: usually a neurosurgeon or an orthopedic surgeon, although there are other kinds of experts in this field.

Diagnosis hinges on many factors, including the great variety of possible causes of back pain and associated symptoms. Most common of these causes is strain of a muscle or a ligament leading to muscle spasm and the painful stiffness that results. In some people emotional tension from anxiety or worry may result in muscle spasm sufficient to cause a stiff, aching back. (These kinds of muscle spasm are usually treated by rest, massage, the local application of heat, diathermy or ultrasound, and medicines that relieve spasm and emotional tension.) Other conditions that must be considered are arthritis, of which there are several kinds; neuritis (inflammation of a nerve); and an unusually loose spinal joint that has allowed slippage of one vertebra on another. Rare afflictions such as a tumor of some sort or abnormal blood vessels of the spine are also possible, although not likely.

How does the specialist determine the exact location and the nature of the trouble?

His first step is careful inquiry into where the pain or other symptoms occur and whether there was any injury or activity that seemed to bring it on. He must also ask whether there have been symptoms of illness elsewhere in the body that might be the cause. This step is called taking the history.

The second step is examination of the patient as a whole and then in detail. Overall examination is designed to rule out evidence of infection, anemia, and serious bodily disease. Detailed tests are then carried out to pinpoint the source of trouble. Clues are points of localized muscle, joint, or nerve tenderness, muscle spasm, and limited motion of the spine, arms, or legs. Muscle power, reflexes, and sensations of various types are then tested to see if they are below par, and if so, exactly where.

The specialist knows exactly where each nerve root of the entire spine is and where each nerve of the body runs. He can therefore tell, on finding something wrong with one, at precisely what spinal level the trouble lies. He knows, for example, that the sciatic nerve, the longest nerve in the body, begins at the lower level of the spine and runs all the way to the toes. Evidence of sciatica, plus other characteristic findings, suggests disc damage in the lowest portion of the spine. Disc rupture in the neck, however, not only may result in nerve-root pain down an arm and other "signature" signs of involvement of that root, but in some cases in compression of the spinal cord. The latter is indicated by weakness and numbness of one or both legs and characteristic abnormalities of leg reflexes.

By this time the history and examination have together supplied a pretty good idea of what and where the trouble is. However, other tests are necessary to be more certain of the diagnosis.

The third diagnostic step, laboratory tests, include appropriate blood tests to rule out infection and other bodily diseases, x-rays of the lungs for the same reason, and x-rays of the suspected area of the spine. The last-mentioned can usually indicate whether a serious type of arthritis exists and what kind of arthritis it is; whether there is any serious slippage of one vertebra on another, or a fracture; and whether by some remote chance there is a spinal tumor of some sort. Because x-rays show bone but not discs, which are mainly cartilage, disc disease can only be surmised on the basis of ordinary spinal x-rays. It may be indicated by the presence of a narrow, instead of a normal, space between two adjacent vertebrae. Narrowing occurs when the disc has ruptured out of the space or has become so degenerated that the uppermost bone has settled down on the one below it.

Sometimes, however, and especially at an early stage in the course of disc trouble, there may not have been sufficient time for a vertebra to settle. In this type of situation the x-rays may therefore appear perfectly normal. Other tests that can be helpful at this stage are electrical tests that show precisely which muscles or nerves are working properly and which are not. The muscle test is called an electromyogram (from the Greek *myo*, muscle) and the other a nerve conduction test. The most reliable and most widely used test, however, is a special procedure known as a myelogram (from *myelo*, spinal).

A myelogram requires a spinal tap for the introduction of a bland liquid, called a contrast fluid because it shows up on x-rays, into the spinal canal. A spinal tap is safe and painless when properly performed. After numbing the skin with local anesthesia, the way a dentist numbs the nerves around a tooth, the doctor gently inserts a small needle into the fluid-filled space inside the lowermost part of the spinal canal, between two vertebral spines. No harm to the spinal cord can occur, because it ends higher up, at the level of the twelfth rib. A teaspoonful or more of the contrast fluid, which resembles pure olive oil, is then introduced through the needle into the spinal canal compartment containing the cerebrospinal fluid. The fluid is opaque to x-rays and therefore can be clearly observed by a fluoroscope and in x-ray films as it is made to flow painlessly up or down inside the spinal canal. It is made to flow, much as mercury is made to shift inside a glass tube, by tilting the patient on an electrically controlled tilt table. The shifting pattern of the contrast material can even be followed on a television screen by a special fluoroscope known as an image-intensifier. This test is used mainly for the detection of a bulging or ruptured disc, or of a spinal tumor, which either stop or simply indent the column of contrast material, depending on their size, at the affected spinal level. Following the test the oil-like liquid is withdrawn.

In my opinion, a myelogram is essential if spinal surgery is contemplated for the removal of a disc or tumor. Otherwise something may be missed—a small benign tumor inside the spinal canal or a disc higher up than the suspected level. This could mean that another operation would have to be performed.

Properly done, a myelogram is seldom painful and it carries virtually no risk. At the same time, it should be said that any such test always carries some risk, however slight. There is, for example, a very remote possibility of nerve-root irritation that could lead to persisting pain, numbness, or weakness, and the equally remote possibility of meningitis, an infection of the CSF. That is why myelograms are not routinely advised when disc trouble is first suspected but are reserved for cases in which pain and perhaps other disability persists despite conservative treatment. Yet in my opinion, the slight risks of the test are more than offset by its value in pinpointing the exact location and nature of the trouble and thus avoiding any unnecessary surgery or a second operation.

How should a suspected or proven damaged disc be treated? If it appears that there is no severe degree of nerve-root pinching and no threat of paralysis of a foot or leg, bed rest for one to six weeks offers a good chance of recovery. The patient should stay in bed the whole time, except possibly for bathroom visits, and not even sit up, as sitting up transfers the weight of the trunk to the offending disc which may bulge out farther or actually rupture.

The person may, however, turn any way he wants in bed. There should be a very firm mattress or a board under the mattress to keep the spine as straight as possible. Points of exquisite local muscle tenderness, called trigger points, may be injected or sprayed with appropriate pain-relieving agents that often allay pain and muscle spasm and contribute to a speedy recovery.

Traction, or steady pulling down of the legs, is believed by some doctors to hasten relief on the theory that traction tends to pull the vertebrae apart just enough to allow the disc to slip back where it belongs. Traction is applied, with the person flat in bed, by means of ankle slings that pass over a pulley to a weight at the foot of the bed. Neck discs may be treated by traction also. The sling in this case fits comfortably around the back of the patient's head and under the chin and is attached to a weight at the head of the bed.

Other non-surgical methods of treatment include efforts to relieve the spasm of back or neck muscles that often occur as the result of disc disease. This is done by massage, the application of heat, and the administration of tranquilizing medicines. In addition, once spasm is relieved, special exercises for the back muscles often strengthen them enough to prevent further disc trouble, as explained in Dr. Hans Kraus's book *The Cause, Prevention and Treatment of Backache, Stress and Tension.*

Sufficient bed rest, with or without traction, will usually cure 80 out of 100 patients whose symptoms have not cleared up spontaneously. For this group, special exercises may then be prescribed to strengthen back muscles and ligaments so that the chance of further disc trouble is lessened. For the remaining 20 percent, surgery offers relief.

Surgery for disc trouble is reserved for those persons whose pain has not cleared up with bed rest or has become recurrent to such an extent that they no longer can or dare engage in normal activities such as sports, travel, and gardening. Surgery is definitely advisable for anyone suffering progressive weakness or actual paralysis of a foot or part of a leg or arm. Otherwise the offending nerve root may become so badly pinched, and for so long a time, that recovery may well be impossible. Evidence of spinal cord compression also calls for prompt surgery.

Disc surgery consists of removing pressure on the nerve root or roots inside the spinal canal by cutting away enough of the lamina, a part of the vertebral arch over the spinal canal, to see the underlying nerve root and remove the disc or any thickened bone beneath it that is the cause of the trouble. Because a lamina, or perhaps parts of two, if two discs are involved, must be partially, but usually not completely, cut away, the operation is known as a laminectomy.

In some clinics orthopedic surgeons perform most or all of these operations. In other clinics they are performed by neurosurgeons, since they are generally more familiar with the course of the nerve roots and nerves involved, especially those in the neck where the spinal cord may also be affected. While surgical decompression of a pinched nerve root is technically a major operation, it is a relatively simple procedure compared with some spinal and most brain operations.

Laminectomy involves the following steps. A skin incision is made directly over the affected portion of the spine. The spinal muscles are then carefully peeled away from their attachments to the appropriate vertebrae so that the lamina of each spinal bone above and below the disc is clearly exposed. A part of each lamina over the disc is then nipped away to create a window in the bone through which the pinched nerve can be seen. A bulging or ruptured disc humps or pushes the nerve root toward the surgeon and usually causes a swollen congested appearance of the root. The latter is now drawn very gently away from the disc beneath it so that the disc can be plainly seen and removed with special instruments. All possible disc material, usually soft and sticky in consistency, is then scraped out from the space between the vertebral bodies with the aim of preventing additional disc fragments from working loose and rupturing at a later date. The nerve root is now free of its previously distorted, pinched, and compressed appearance. The muscles and skin are then stitched together to finish the operation.

After disc surgery most patients are encouraged to get out of bed a day or so later and are usually able to leave the hospital in six to ten days. They then take things easy at home for a week or so and return to work by easy stages, depending on their disposition, well-being, and the nature of their work. The ultimate outlook for permanent recovery is generally excellent, although there are certain exceptions.

One is the ever-present, although very rare, possibility that some fragment of a disc, which could not be removed despite every effort, will work loose at a later date and again pinch the nerve root. This eventuality requires a second operation, usually simpler than the first because the bone window in the spine has already been made at the first operation.

Another complication that may develop is low-back pain after disc removal. This occurs in some persons because their spinal joints are either exceptionally loose or arthritic, or because the vertebral bones have settled so much that their joints grind together and thus cause pain. In this respect it should be emphasized that the vertebra above a damaged disc, whether the disc is removed or is left in place without surgery, tends to settle on the bone below it. Most people, however, do not experience much or any pain as the result of this settling, despite narrowing of the normal disc space. There are many people, including the writer, who, because of long-past accidents in sports, have practically no lumbar disc spaces left and yet have no back or leg pains whatsoever.

If low-back pain does occur and persist after disc surgery, it can usually be corrected by an operation known as a spinal fusion. With the idea of preventing this type of low-back pain, many orthopedic surgeons advocate spinal fusion at the time of disc surgery. Spinal fusion at the time of lumbar disc surgery is also advocated by orthopedic surgeons in the belief that discs bulge or rupture because the adjacent spinal joints are so loose that they permit an excessive degree of motion of the vertebrae, imposing an extra strain on the disc and its ligaments so that it bulges and ruptures. On the presumption that a loose joint has caused the disc trouble in the first place, it is therefore argued that the joint or joints should be made solid by fusion.

Undoubtedly this theory applies to some disc cases; but in my opinion spinal fusion is not indicated in every disc case. However, I do believe that it is clearly indicated when special tests show that the affected spinal joints are so loose as to cause low-back pain.

What is a spinal fusion? In essence it means "welding" part of the spine with bone grafts to strengthen it. Bone for the grafts may be taken from the hip, which has plenty of bone to spare, or may be banked bone, of which there are several varieties. The surgeon who performs the fusion chooses the bone for a graft and the precise manner in which it is used.

A highly effective and safe method of decompressing pinched nerve roots in the neck and then fusing that part of the neck is by making an incision in the front of the neck. Disc material can then be well removed from between two vertebrae and the bony opening sealed with a peg-shaped bone graft. After this type of operation patients usually get out of bed promptly and go back to work in a few days.

While spinal fusion in the lumbar level is generally effective in 95 percent of the cases and does not limit normal athletic or other activities, I do not favor its routine use for several reasons. First, it makes a disc operation appreciably longer, and it is an age-old surgical axiom that the longer any operation, the greater are the chances for complications. Second, it sometimes leads to disc rupture at the next higher level of the spine. This is because it welds two vertebrae solidly together and thus transfers most of the spinal stresses and strains to the next higher level, where ligaments and the disc take such a beating that disc rupture eventually may occur. My third and most serious objection to routine fusions of the lumbar, though not to the neck, region of the spine, is that an average of two transfusions of blood is usually necessary. Despite every modern precaution it is still possible, even though it is extremely rare, for a transfusion to lead to serum hepatitis, a potentially very serious liver disease.

Every patient should be fully apprised of the various risks relating to myelography, disc surgery, and spinal fusion, together with the benefits that each offers. Fortunately the benefits by far outweigh the very slight risks.

To sum up, a person first afflicted with low-back pain should not be alarmed, because the probability is that he simply has muscle spasm that will go away with conservative treatment. Should there be leg pain in addition to backache, disc damage may then be suspected. But again, conservative treatment, as outlined, usually provides reasonably prompt and often lasting relief, especially if followed by appropriate exercises designed to strengthen the back and prevent recurrent symptoms. If disability continues, is severe, and prevents normal activities, then a myelogram is indicated, after other simpler tests have been made, to see whether or not a suspected disc is really the cause of the trouble. If it is, disc surgery offers a splendid chance of lasting relief. Spinal fusion at the time of disc surgery is theoretically a good idea, for a patient with a successfully fused spine is practically guaranteed against further trouble at that location. However, for the reasons cited, it is my belief that routine spinal fusion at the time of disc surgery is not always indicated, especially as it can always be performed at a later date should the need arise.

Advances in the Field

A substance has recently been found that softens and practically dissolves the discs of the spine, according to a recent report by Dr. Bernard Sussman of Washington, D.C. Although it is still in the experimental stage, it holds the promise of softening slipped discs when injected into them. It is a substance related to papain, a ferment of pawpaw fruit, which can tenderize meat and if given to rabbits make their ears so floppy they won't stand up! This treatment, if it stands the test of time, may be a cure for associated sciatica without the need of disc surgery.

Another and quite spectacular advance in chemical treatment concerns a bone condition called Paget's disease after the British physician, Sir James Paget, who described it approximately 100 years ago. It is a thickening of bone of unknown cause, which can affect practically any bone of the body. When it affects the spine, the thickened bone can squeeze nerve roots or even the spinal cord itself and cause serious symptoms, including paralysis of the legs (paraplegia) and pain resembling that caused by a slipped disc. Some textbooks as recently as 1970 state that there is no effective treatment other than surgery to remove the diseased bone that is pressing on the spinal cord. Yet today, only a short time later, three substances have been found that prevent progression of the disease. One of these can lead to harmful side effects, while another often ceases to be effective after six months or so, but the third has so far seemed perfectly harmless and remarkably effective. Surprisingly enough, it is actually a detergent for removing calcium scales from metal pipes! Its use for treating Paget's disease was based on scientific detective work, too complicated to describe briefly, which suggested that it might also be useful for remedying certain bone disorders accompanied by disturbances in calcium and also phosphorus metabolism. Trials of one to two years' duration have shown that it can arrest the progressive bone thickening of Paget's disease, promote bone healing, and restore associated abnormalities of blood chemistry to normal.

2

Nerve
and Spinal
Injuries

Nerve Fibers

The nervous system is a vast communications complex. It is composed of billions of nerve cells that send and receive all the messages, or signals, that travel along delicate filaments, called nerve fibers, to other nerve cells or various parts of the body. It is a system that literally extends from head to toe and is essential for our survival and actions. As already mentioned, the nervous system consists of three principal parts: the brain, the spinal cord, and the nerves. The brain and spinal cord together are called the central nervous system, while the nerves of the body are known as peripheral nerves (in contrast to the nerves of the brain, which are called cranial nerves).

All the information reaching the brain, whether it concerns the outside world or internal feelings such as hunger or pain, depends on special kinds of nerve cells that are sensitive to specific changes in their environment. While the human body contains millions of these sensory cells, there are special varieties, different in cellular size, shape, and microscopic appearance, for each kind of sensation. One type of cell, for example, is exclusively reserved for the detection of skin temperature, while another variety registers only postural changes in muscles.

Each sensory cell consists of a central body with a threadlike filament, called a nerve fiber, or axon, reaching out from it. Nerves are formed by merged nerve fibers.

In addition to these sensory fibers, most nerves of the body also contain motor fibers. These are outgrowths of nerve cells in the spinal cord, whose function is to make something happen: to make a muscle move or a gland become active. A nerve, therefore, is not an isolated unit of the body, like a bone, but represents groups of nerve fibers that are all extensions or continuations of nerve cells.

All nerve signals originate in a nerve cell called a neuron and are a result of weak electrical charges with simultaneous chemical changes that then travel along the nerve fibers at high speeds.

Each kind of information from the body goes, in the form of nerve signals, to a special part of the brain, and only when the message arrives do you feel a touch, a change of temperature, or become aware of the position of your arm or leg. Somehow the brain registers these small electro-chemical changes as meaningful patterns of each variety of sensation. But when a nerve is badly damaged, this system of delicate communication partly breaks down. The result is numbness and muscle weakness or paralysis because messages can no longer travel along the nerve, past the point of injury, to reach the muscles supplied by that nerve.

Injured Nerves

As an example of what happens when an important nerve is injured, consider the following case.

Mr. V., a lanky young engineer, recently came to my office, terribly worried because his right foot had become numb and partly paralyzed. It had been so for a week. Questioning, confirmed by my examination, indicated that the top of his foot was numb, and that he could not lift either the toes or the foot. The foot simply flopped like a dead fish when he walked—a condition known as foot drop.

The muscles that were paralyzed and the area of skin that was numb are both supplied by one nerve, a branch of the sciatic called the peroneal nerve. Knowing this, I asked him if he could possibly have injured his right knee in any way, for the most likely point of an injury to this nerve is at the outer side of the knee, directly below the joint. At this spot, the peroneal nerve twines around the outermost of the two leg bones, just under the skin, where it can easily be injured and cause his type of numbness and paralysis.

"Yes," he said, "I know exactly how the trouble might have started, because I noticed that my foot was numb and weak the moment I stood up in a theater after watching a long movie. For the last hour or so of the movie my legs were stretched over the two empty seats in front of me, and I remember distinctly that my right knee had slipped into the V between two chair backs, where it was sort of wedged in. Could this have caused the trouble?"

I assured him that I thought so, that the peroneal had been pressed upon by the chair long enough to damage it. I added that he definitely did not have a slipped disc, which he had thought was the trouble, and that he would regain full use of the foot. Since this would probably take quite a while, I prescribed a foot-drop brace to keep the paralyzed muscles from being over-stretched and physiotherapy to speed muscle recovery. I also explained that this type of nerve injury is well known, especially in thin, lanky persons who do not have much fat between the skin and the nerve to protect the nerve from pressure. Thin persons may even develop a foot drop from keeping their legs crossed in a position that causes pressure upon this nerve by the opposite knee.

As another example of this type of nerve injury, but one which affects the hand, I mentioned "Saturday night palsy," a condition which occasionally afflicts persons subject to over-indulgence in alcohol. They fall asleep with one arm over the back of a chair and wake up on Sunday morning unable to lift the hand or straighten out the fingers of that arm. The lifting muscles have become paralyzed because the radial nerve, one of the three main arm nerves, has been temporarily rendered functionless. It has been compressed in the armpit, through which the nerve passes.

When Mr. V. asked how long it would take for his foot to stage a full recovery, I replied that it might take three to four months. Upset by this, he pressed for an explanation of why it would take so long. I took time to explain in considerable detail what nerves are like and why recovery may be slow after a nerve has been badly injured. I began by saying that nerves constitute the wiring system of the body, and they are made up of many individually insulated filaments, like the wires of a cable, called nerve fibers. Every major nerve of the body contains two principal kinds of nerve fibers: sensory fibers, which carry messages of sensation, and motor fibers, which carry messages from the brain and spinal cord that activate and control muscles and other body functions. If the sensory fibers are knocked out by injury or disease, numbness will result, and if the motor fibers are damaged, there will be paralysis of the muscles and other structures which the nerve supplies.

I added that nerves are pretty well protected from the stresses and strains of everyday life because all their delicate fibers are enclosed within a fairly tough outer envelope of tissue, called a nerve sheath, and also because most nerves of the body, except at a few points, are sandwiched between muscles, which protect them from injury. In addition, nerves have a rubbery consistency that makes them flexible enough to withstand motions such as the bending of joints.

I then pointed out that three things can happen when a nerve is injured, depending on how severe the injury has been. A very light blow directly over a nerve, for example, not hard enough to cause any permanent damage, may simply send a shower of signals up the nerve. These signals reach the spinal cord, where all nerves of the body terminate, and are relayed to the brain, where they are registered as painful, tingling sensations. They occur because the sensory fibers of the nerve have been stimulated by the blow, which, crudely speaking, results in a sort of internal "sparking" that gives rise to too many signals.

If you have ever banged your elbow, I continued, and felt a tingling sensation shoot down to your little finger, you have suffered such a nerve injury. The shock sensation occurs because you have struck the ulnar nerve, one of the three main nerves of your arm, where it is most vulnerable to injury—just before it enters a groove (which you can feel) in the so-called funny bone. The tingling is caused by striking, not the bone, but the nerve, as you can discover for yourself. Tap the bone sharply with a finger tip and no tingling results. But tap directly over the nerve, either just above or within the bony groove, and you can then elicit a brief "funny bone" shock. This commonplace phenomenon illustrates how sensitive a nerve is.

Should this nerve be struck very sharply, it could be put out of commission for a matter of several minutes or even hours. The result would be numbness and partial paralysis of the little finger and adjacent part of the hand, which depend on the ulnar nerve for sensation and the ability to move some of the gripping muscles. This condition represents a nerve concussion, which is similar to a brain concussion. It is somewhat like a local short circuit that prevents any signals from passing the point of injury. There is recovery because there has been no permanent damage. But recovery may take several hours or days if the blow has resulted in any congestion, or local nerve swelling, for this will prevent the passage of signals. Not until the swelling subsides will the nerve again function normally.

The third thing that can happen is prolonged numbness and paralysis ("which I fear you are in for," I said to Mr. V.) because of a really severe nerve injury. Such an injury, whether from compression, bruising, or actual cutting of a nerve, has two effects. First, it destroys the delicate nerve fibers at the point of injury. Second, it causes the entire length of each damaged fiber to disintegrate or wither away all the way down to the skin and muscles that the nerve supplies—a phenomenon known as nerve degeneration. If the damaged nerve has not been cut, recovery can take place. But this takes time, because recovery depends on a regrowth of nerve fibers from the point of injury to their usual destination. This regrowth, known as nerve regeneration, takes place because the healthy intact nerve fibers immediately above the point of injury sprout new fibers. Since sprouting proceeds at a rate of only one to two millimeters (about one sixteenth of an inch) a day, it takes a long time for each reconstituted fiber to reach its destination and again transmit messages to and from the spinal cord and brain.

"Another question, Doctor—supposing my leg nerve doesn't recover. What then?"

I replied that it might then be necessary to operate and repair the nerve, just as if it had been cut. There seemed little chance that he would need an operation, but in some cases the injury is so severe that it leads to scar formation in or around a nerve. The scar tissue obstructs the regrowth of sprouting nerve fibers and makes recovery impossible. The formation of a thick wall of scar tissue between two ends of a nerve that has been severed is also a reason why cut nerves do not recover. Still another reason is that the two ends tend to pull apart, because of the natural elasticity of nerves. Therefore even if sprouting fibers succeed in growing through or around the intervening scar tissue, they usually fail to find their way into the other end of the cut nerve.

The young man finally departed, and eventually regained full use of his paralyzed foot without requiring a nerve repair. But some are not as fortunate, as illustrated by the next two cases.

All five fingers of the left hand of a talented pianist became paralyzed by a nerve injury so severe that he literally could not lift a finger—or even his hand. One of the three main nerves to the hand, the radial, had been cut by a deep gash in the arm suffered during an automobile accident. Without surgical repair of the nerve his career as a pianist would have tragically ended. A year after nerve surgery he was playing the piano again.

A lad of 15, young R., was run over by a steel runner of a sled, which sliced his sciatic nerve in two just above the right knee. His foot immediately became paralyzed and flopped, like Mr. V.'s, when he tried to walk. Six months after nerve repair there was scarcely a trace of weakness or of the foot numbness that had also occurred. Four years later he became a fighter pilot. He told me that the Air Force physicians who examined him found it hard to believe the nerve had ever been injured.

In each of these cases the injury occurred at the exact location of a nerve. Had the gash or cut been half an inch to either side, the nerve would not have been touched.

A nerve tumor may also interrupt the function of a nerve. Nerve tumors are rare and very seldom malignant.

They can be surgically removed by cutting across the nerve at each end of the tumor and sewing the two ends together, as in nerve repair.

Parenthetically, a promising new method of finding out how badly a nerve is damaged is by means of an ultra-sensitive device for detecting the miniscule magnetic currents that emanate from healthy nerves. It is a device similar in principle to that used for geodetic surveys and the detection of hidden ores by aerial survey. With this apparatus held close to the skin, it is now possible to detect the very faint magnetic fields of nerves of the body and tell whether they are functioning normally or are cut or diseased.

Surgical Nerve Repair

Repair of a severly injured nerve requires an operation to remove the damaged segment of nerve by cutting it cleanly across, just above and just below the mangled portion. The two healthy ends of the nerve are then sewn together, end-to-end, by tiny stitches passed through their sheath. Repair is facilitated because of the nerve's elasticity, which permits enough stretching to bring the two cut ends together after an injured segment has been removed. Recovery after repair of a major nerve of an arm or leg takes time because new nerve fibers grow down the nerve so very slowly.

In addition to arm, leg, and even small finger nerves, it is sometimes possible to repair the nerves that move the muscles of the face. When one of these has been permanently put out of commission by an inflammation, an injury, or a tumor, that side of the face droops in an unsightly, expressionless fashion. This kind of paralysis, involving one entire side of the face including the forehead muscles, is called Bell's palsy, after a famous Scottish neurologist

Sir Charles Bell (1774–1842). (The facial weakness caused by a stroke or other kinds of brain damage, which cannot be repaired, does not paralyze the forehead muscles nor does it completely paralyze all facial movements as Bell's palsy does.)

If congestion is the cause of the paralysis, Bell's palsy may be cured by ear surgery to remove bone surrounding the facial nerve and relieve pressure on the nerve. In some cases it is even possible to replace a damaged portion of the nerve with a nerve graft to restore function. Certain other cases require a neurosurgical operation that involves stitching a healthy nerve in the neck to the paralyzed facial nerve. The "donor" nerve most frequently used for this purpose is that which moves the corresponding half of the tongue. Control of that side of the tongue, but not of the other side, will of course be reduced, but not sufficiently to prevent useful speech or swallowing. When nerve fibers from the tongue nerve have grown down the facial nerve to the muscles of the face, control of facial motion and expression is regained by thinking of moving the tongue. In time, facial expressions and movements generally become automatic. Still another way of correcting facial palsy is by plastic surgery.

For all the advances in modern neurosurgery, there are nonetheless certain repairs that cannot be made. Sometimes, for example, I have been asked why vision cannot be restored to a blind eye by repairing the optic, or vision, nerve. The reason is that the optic nerve is not a true nerve. It is simply an extension of brain tissue, which, once badly damaged, can never be repaired.

More often I have been asked whether persisting numbness of the skin around the scar of any operation can be corrected or is a sign of trouble. The answer to both questions is no. The numbness is not a sign of trouble. It simply occurs because any incision must cut through some of the nerves for sensation and thus lead to numbness.

Permanent numbness may also be caused, although rarely, by a Novocain block of a jaw nerve, as for a tooth extraction, or as a result of the extraction itself. This can happen, through no fault of the dentist, because the injection has resulted in a tiny hemorrhage inside the nerve that deadens it, or because the extraction has torn the nerve. Because the nerve is so small and in such an inaccessible place, any attempt to repair it would probably fail, in contrast to larger, accessible nerves like those of an arm or leg, which can usually be repaired with success.

Injuries to the Spine

Single nerves lend themselves to repair in large part because they are fairly simple structures compared to the spinal cord, which is not. Nerves from all over the body feed into this cable of the brain, which contains not only nerve fibers but also nerve cells that relay all messages to and from the brain. Obviously, therefore, if the spinal cord is injured, many nerves will be affected, because they can then neither receive messages from the brain nor send their sensory or informational messages to it. Consequently, paralysis and numbness may occur in one leg (monoplegia), both legs (paraplegia), or even all four limbs (quadriplegia), in contrast to the paralysis of only a few muscles and the numbness of only a relatively small area of the body that a nerve injury may cause.

Fortunately, the spinal cord is not always permanently injured by an accident. It may have been only temporarily put out of commission by a relatively minor jolt or sudden stretching that results in spinal-cord concussion, similar to concussion of the brain, from which complete recovery can take place. I have seen this happen after a so-called whiplash injury of the neck.

In this instance, I heard the screech of brakes and a

crash just outside my home. When I dashed out to the road, I found that a sports car had rammed into the rear of a small sedan. The driver of the sports car was uninjured, but the young man driving the sedan remained seated at the wheel, unable to move because both legs were paralyzed and numb. His hands were also slightly weak and numb. Perfectly rational, he complained of pain in the neck and said that his head and neck had been snapped backward, whereupon his legs immediately became numb and limp. By the time an ambulance arrived, about fifteen minutes later, he had recovered full power and sensation in his legs and arms. X-rays at the local hospital showed no evidence of a spinal fracture or of displacement of a vertebra. A week later the young man returned to work and has remained free of symptoms.

More severe spinal injuries usually lead to symptoms that do not clear up. But there are a few such injuries that can be corrected, with relief of paralysis and numbness. These are pressure injuries, in which there is just enough pressure against the spinal cord to prevent the transmission of nerve signals, but not enough to have cut or otherwise permanently damaged the cord. Pressure injuries, for example, may be caused by a spent bullet that happens to lodge next to the cord without permanently damaging it. I have succeeded in relieving paralysis and numbness in the legs in a few such cases, while working in an Army field hospital during World War II, by removing the bullet or shell fragment that had been pressing on the cord, or a fragment of bone, shattered by the missile, that had been driven up against the cord, and occasionally a sizable blood clot caused by a wound close to the spine.

The most common correctable type of spinal injury that has led to weakness and numbness of the limbs is a dislocation, or slippage, of one vertebra on another, such that the spinal cord is pinched but not seriously damaged. Here is an example.

A boy of fourteen, young D., while catching behind home plate, was run into by a runner from third base. The runner dashed at full speed against the young catcher's head, which was jarred abruptly backward. Young D. immediately crumpled to the ground and could not get up because his legs were paralyzed. He was promptly brought to a local hospital where I saw him at once. By this time he was able to move his legs a little, although they were still dreadfully weak, and he complained of pain high up in the neck. On examination I found that the leg and arm reflexes were not normal—indicating spinal cord trouble high in the neck—and that his legs were numb. X-rays showed a frightening-looking backward displacement of the uppermost vertebra of the neck. It was clear that his head had been so badly jarred that this vertebra had suffered a serious dislocation, which was compressing the spinal cord.

Treatment, which was carried out at once, consisted of a procedure known as cervical (neck) tong traction. This meant the application of a pair of metal tongs, similar in appearance to those used for carrying large blocks of ice. The tip of each tong is very easily and painlessly inserted into a tiny hole made part way through the bone at each side of the skull. This requires only a very small incision in the scalp on each side, after injecting the scalp with a little Novocain. A weight is then attached to the tongs to pull on the head and thus straighten out the deformity in the neck. Within thirty minutes D. regained considerable power and sensation in his legs, and by this time an abnormal toe reflex, a danger sign which had been present, had disappeared. X-rays now showed perfectly straight, normal-looking neck bones. The dislocation had been corrected, or, technically speaking, reduced. A cast was applied to his neck to prevent recurrence of the slippage until healing took place, and he recovered all the lost spinal-cord functions completely.

Sometimes the effects of a spinal injury are far more devastating, but nevertheless correctable to some degree by a combination of traction and spinal surgery. I am thinking now of a beautiful, talented young woman, Miss J., who was a victim of a terrible head-on automobile collision. She was found in her overturned sports car, completely helpless because of total paralysis from the neck down, and was carefully removed from the car by three men of the well-trained volunteer ambulance crew. This care in moving her was probably a major reason why she eventually recovered as well as she did.

(If you happen to be at the scene of an accident, the essential thing to know is that most injuries of the spine in ordinary life cause or threaten paralysis because the spinal cord is pinched either by a vertebra that has been dislocated or by a fragment of bone from a fractured vertebra. The victim should not be hastily or carelessly moved, for this could make a dislocation worse or further dislodge a piece of fractured bone, thus converting a possibly minor degree of spinal-cord damage into one from which there can be no hope of recovery. To avoid this risk, the victim's spine should be kept as straight as possible and never bent. And it is advisable to move the person with the aid of at least three people in order to prevent buckling of the spine that could permanently damage the cord.)

As soon as Miss J. arrived at the hospital, x-rays were taken that showed a mild degree of dislocation of a lower neck vertebra. Traction was therefore instituted, as in the boy's case, and in a few days there were signs of some return of sensation and recovery—a little leg and arm motion, but no finger motion. Suspecting the possibility of a slipped disc in the neck, which is sometimes also present with this type of injury, I arranged a myelogram. Because it did reveal that a disc was pressing on the spinal cord, I operated to remove the disc and relieve the pressure. Thereafter she slowly and steadily improved, although never regaining full use of her arm, hand, and leg muscles. For three months she had to be kept in a special bed called a Stryker frame, in order to maintain neck traction and permit easy turning of her body from front to back every few hours to avoid bedsores of the skin.

Meanwhile, daily exercises and massage were prescribed to speed the recovery of muscle power. But her own courage and determination were key factors in her recovery. Miss J. made constant efforts to develop the strength of whatever muscles she was able to move, even though at first she could only make them twitch feebly. This is one of the most important things a person can do to help any weak muscles regain power. The more that voluntary efforts are made to exercise them, the better are the chances for their recovery.

At the end of six months she was able to use the typewriter, although painfully slowly, and to walk with special (Canadian) crutches. Slow improvement continued during the ensuing six months, until, a year after her accident and almost total paralysis, she was able to drive her car wherever she wanted, with the aid of special fittings for the gear shift and brakes. She has since married and leads an extremely active and constructive life, in spite of having to use her crutches. Complete recovery did not take place because part of the spinal cord remained irreparably damaged.

The fact that very weak and even withered muscles can be restored to full strength, with diligent exercise, is dramatically illustrated by some victims of poliomyelitis. Two outstanding examples are a former figure skating champion and a well-known track star. Both had suffered a marked degree of leg paralysis when very young, which they were determined to overcome by exercise and hard work to develop their weak withered muscles!

The muscles do not necessarily wither away solely because they cannot be moved and therefore exercised.

Another reason may be damage to the trophic fibers of a nerve—those that govern the metabolism and growth of tissues, including muscles.

As the cases cited earlier illustrate, the cord is highly vulnerable to injury. There are three principal reasons. First, the spinal cord is very small in comparison with its tremendous importance. It is only about three-quarters of an inch in diameter, and yet it carries almost all nerve messages between the brain and the body. Even a small injury to it can therefore wreak great havoc. Second, it is confined within and practically fills a very small space, the bony canal of the spine. The addition of anything else, such as dislocated or fractured bone, a ruptured disc, or the inward buckling of a spinal ligament, can very easily pinch or bruise the cord so badly that it ceases to function. Third, if badly damaged, the spinal cord, unlike a nerve, cannot establish effective new nerve connections by regeneration, nor can it ever be repaired by surgery or any other means.

Too often severe spinal injuries lead to permanent paralysis of both legs, or both arms as well as both legs, and in addition, abolish bladder and bowel control as well as sexual potency, and lead to complete numbness of the body below the level of the injury. This is all the more tragic because war wounds in young soldiers and automobile accidents in young civilians account for many cases of paraplegia and quadriplegia in the very prime of life—the worst time for a loss of sexual potency and the crippling that interrupts a promising career.

The sooner rehabilitation efforts by physiotherapy are started, the better. Massage and exercises, which should be prescribed and directed by an expert, can often prevent temporarily paralyzed or partly paralyzed muscles from wasting away, which they are apt to do. In addition, physiotherapy helps prevent stiffening of the joints. If not all of the back muscles have been paralyzed, paraplegic persons can even learn to walk with the aid of special braces and crutches. Treatment also includes constant efforts to avoid skin sores and bladder and other infections, to which paraplegics are extremely susceptible. And if severe spasms of the legs occur, they can be relieved by medical or surgical treatment.

New Developments in Treatment

Some of the most fascinating and exciting new discoveries concern the prevention of dangerously severe swelling of the spinal cord—the kind that threatens paralysis—after it has been partly crushed by an injury.

A blow to the spinal cord soon causes it to swell from rapidly spreading local congestion. Laboratory tests I have recently heard of indicate that this rapidly spreading congestion is caused in large part by chemical chain reactions affecting the spinal cord's cells and even the tiny blood vessels inside the spinal cord. Swelling and hemorrhage can occur as a result of the chemical changes in the spinal cord. If they persist, the nerve cells and fibers of the cord can be permanently destroyed.

Additional experiments have shown that these reactions can be slowed or stopped by certain chemical agents provided they are administered soon after the cord injury. Trials of these agents have already shown that animals that would otherwise be permanently paraplegic quickly recover and soon walk about as nimbly and normally as if their spinal cord had never been injured. This is because serious spinal cord swelling had been prevented. Exactly the same type of injury led to permanent paraplegia in animals which were not treated with these agents.

This work suggests that perhaps prompt (even roadside) treatment of persons with severe spinal injuries might prevent the cord swelling that so often is the cause of permanent paraplegia.

Other tests on animals indicate that local cooling of the damaged portion of the spinal cord, if done within two to three hours after the injury, can prevent the permanent paraplegia that afflicts other animals subjected to an equivalent injury but not given the cooling treatment. It remains to be shown, however, whether this technique will prove either safe or effective for treating a badly injured spinal cord in human beings, especially as an operation is required to expose the damaged portion of the cord in order to cool it with an ice-cold saline solution.

There is even a dream of someday being able to help the paraplegic regain at least some ability to walk by finding out how to promote regrowth (regeneration) of damaged nerve fibers in the spinal cord, or by wiring the spinal cord or its nerve roots so that signals from the brain or from healthy nerves can be transmitted to portions of the cord which have been isolated by an injury. This wiring project would require a unit provided with many fine wires, a miniature computer, and a tiny long-lasting battery placed permanently under the skin, near the spine. Such a device has already been designed and constructed. It is a compact unit only about an inch square and is a side result of the miniaturization of computers and other electronic devices perfected for space craft. Such a device is comparable to, although more complicated than, the pacemakers placed in the body for the regulation of the heart rate. A somewhat similar device has already been developed by Dr. Blain Nashold of Duke University, to provide artificial bladder control in paraplegic patients. This device electrically stimulates the lowermost part of the spinal cord—called the conus because of its cone shape —where the bladder nerves originate. When these nerves are electrically stimulated, they cause contraction of muscles that empty the bladder. Whether these devices will prove effective in the long run remains to be seen.

But regardless of these developments, efforts to restore lost functions and to preserve all possible intact functions depends on rehabilitation therapy. It is a tremendous tribute to the courage of most paraplegics and some quadriplegics that they learn to conquer their disability and continue to lead productive and active lives. For example, a paraplegic person, even if he cannot manage brace and crutch walking, can lead a remarkably active wheelchair existence.

Injuries to the nervous system have in recent years increased so rapidly that committees have been established to study the kinds of accidents that result in such injuries, means of reducing such accidents, and ways of improving medical and surgical treatment. In addition, considerable research is being conducted in this and other countries to study details of nerve, spinal-cord, and brain injuries in an effort to understand them better so that they can be treated more effectively. Finally, as described in a later chapter, miniature computers and electrical circuits are being developed that may some day artificially restore control to paralyzed muscles. Thus there is considerable hope for the future.

3

Skull
and Brain
Injuries

The Protective Skull

While the skull has long been a symbol of death, as in the skull and crossbones of the pirates' Jolly Roger, poor Yorick's skull in *Hamlet*, and its use on bottles of deadly poison, in the eyes of a brain surgeon it is a benevolent guardian. The skull is a bony helmet that provides protection and support for that mysterious mass of soft tissue, the human brain. Without the skull we would all be vulnerable to concussion and other brain injuries from even the slightest jolts and jarrings.

The structural growth of the skull is one of nature's most beautiful feats of engineering. In the newborn baby, as every parent knows, the skull is not yet hard, but soft and rubbery, being formed then only of islands of cartilagelike tissue that are not solid bone. This provides an elasticity that makes delivery of the infant easier for the mother and allows for the growth of the brain. This resilience also explains why a baby may fall from his crib and bump his head without harm. Even if his head strikes an object, the soft skull will not crack, as an adult skull may, but will only be bent inward the way a ping-pong ball is dented.

As a child grows, the soft thin rubbery islands of the skull gradually grow larger, thicker, and harder until finally the spaces between them fill with solid bone that welds them together. Not only do these bone islands come to fit as neatly as the pieces of a jigsaw puzzle, but they also become locked in place by myriads of tiny teeth lining their edges. These teeth on each piece of bone mesh with those of adjoining bones, like the teeth of joining gears, and then become solidly fused by calcification, providing structural reinforcement. The solidification process, however, is not complete until a person is approximately twenty-one years old.

Skull Fractures

A skull fracture is not necessarily serious, although the term is frightening to the layman. A fracture is even protective when enough of the force of a head injury is taken by the skull to prevent damage to the brain. Under these circumstances the head can be compared with an egg, whose shell can be cracked or fractured without injury to the yolk inside.

The simplest kind of skull fracture is called a linear fracture because it appears on x-rays as a fairly straight line. A prominent surgeon sustained just such a fracture recently while skiing. Falling sharply on the back of his head, he was momentarily dazed but never unconscious. There was no cut on the scalp, and no reflex or other changes on examination to indicate any brain damage, although x-rays showed a fracture line at the back of the skull. After a few days of bed rest, during which he felt a little groggy and suffered some headache, he felt perfectly well, and resumed his usual schedule of operating a week after the injury. Like other linear fractures, this one healed by itself.

Linear fractures can be dangerous, however, if the crack crosses just in front of the ear and the major bone artery there is torn. A large hemorrhage inside the skull may occur so rapidly and result in so much pressure on the brain that the brain cannot function and the person may die within the hour unless brain surgery is performed. The first case of this kind that I treated was a young man, Mr. L., who had had a bad motorcycle accident and was brought to the hospital in a state of unconsciousness. X-rays showed a fracture line crossing the path of the bone artery in front of his right ear, which immediately suggested the possibility of a serious hemorrhage from this vessel. The operating room was at once prepared. By the time the x-rays had been developed, the patient had briefly regained consciousness and was able to talk. A few minutes afterward, however, he lapsed again into unconsciousness—a sign typical of these hemorrhages.

Surgery was promptly performed. Through a small opening in the bone at the right temple directly over the fracture line, the clot was removed and the bleeding stopped. The operation was carried out under local (Novocain) anesthesia only, and before the last stitch had been tied, the patient was already beginning to wake up. Mr. L. enjoyed a rapid and perfect recovery, but had surgery been delayed, he would not have survived.

Another possible complication of some linear fractures is leakage of cerebrospinal fluid from the nose or ear. This can happen if the fracture extends into one of the cavities or sinuses of the skull that contain air, like the frontal sinuses of the forehead, which communicate with the nasal passages. It can also happen if the crack enters the mastoid air cells behind the ear, at the base of the skull, for then CSF can leak out the ear if the eardrum has also been ruptured by the injury, as often happens. Danger lies in the fact that if CSF leaks out, bacteria may find their way into the head and cause meningitis. Fortunately most leaking fractures of these varieties heal themselves so that the leakage stops. Persons having such a leak are treated by absolute rest in bed, with the head elevated to reduce the fluid pressure inside it and thus minimize the outflow of liquid. Antibiotics are given to prevent meningitis. If the leak does not stop after a week or so, surgery is advisable to seal the crack in the bone with a small piece of muscle or a plastic substance that hardens quickly like a glue.

Any fracture in which bone has been exposed to the outside by a break in the scalp or skin is called a compound fracture. Because the scalp has such a rich supply of blood, even a small cut, whether or not it is associated with a fracture, will usually lead to profuse bleeding. Although blood in the hair, and perhaps also streaming down over the face, gives the victim a frightening appearance, it is reassuring to know that firm pressure, preferably with a clean cloth, will slow or stop the bleeding until a doctor can treat the wound. There is no danger to the brain from a simple scalp cut, provided that it is properly and promptly managed and there is no fracture, since the scalp's blood vessels do not nourish the brain.

My experience in war surgery and various city hospitals has shown, surprisingly enough, that compound fractures from bullet, knife, or other injuries may be sustained without even causing loss of consciousness. I vividly remember a young man, Mr. P., on whom I operated years ago to remove a steel rod that had pierced his skull from top to bottom but merely dazed him. He had been walking home from work when a steel rod, six feet long and half an inch in diameter, fell from the third story of a construction project. Before bringing him to the hospital, the police emergency squad had to cut off all but a protruding six inches of the rod in order to get him inside the ambulance.

On arrival at the hospital Mr. P. was remarkably calm and suffering no pain or other symptoms. The piece of rod was sticking straight up from his head, just back of the hairline, in a line directly above his right eye. I could feel the lower end of the rod just under the skin at the angle of his right jaw. X-rays of course showed the rod and also showed two small circular fractures around it, one where it had pierced the top of the head, and the other at the base of the skull.

Removal of the rod was tricky, because its inner portion was only an eighth of an inch away from the large bone artery at the base of the skull. Simply pulling the rod out could easily have ripped this artery and resulted in fatal hemorrhage. The first order of business was, therefore, an operation to seal off the artery at the base of the skull. It was then a simple matter to carry out a second operation at the top of the head in order to remove bone that was wedging the rod in place. The rod was then gently and readily pulled out. Before the scalp was stitched up, the wound was thoroughly cleansed, a procedure known as debridement, by trimming off jagged edges of bone and injured scalp and flushing the wound copiously with a saline solution.

The patient made a perfect recovery. His lack of symptoms is explained by the fact that the injury to the right frontal lobe, which had been penetrated by the rod, was neither large enough to cause any symptoms nor in a location that could lead to paralysis. It was not, moreover, the kind of injury that jars the brain as a whole, as do most other kinds of head injury.

The forward portion of either the right or left temporal lobe is particularly vulnerable to penetrating injuries by a knife blade, ice pick, or other small, sharp object, for the bone over this area is unusually thin compared with the rest of the skull. Like the forward portion of either frontal lobe, the forward portion of either temporal lobe, as I have frequently seen, can also sustain a penetrating injury, provided it is not a large one, without serious symptoms. This is because these portions of the frontal and temporal lobes do not contain nerve cells or connecting fibers whose damage can lead to paralysis or to any other disability except possible temporary alteration in emotional control and emotional reactions—usually in the direction of euphoria, or inappropriate cheerfulness. The reason permanent or marked emotional alterations do not as a rule occur following comparatively minor injuries to one of these parts of the brain is that the opposite frontal or temporal lobe and the remainder of the injured lobe are capable of carrying on a normal degree of emotional control.

The patient with a bullet in his brain raises several questions for the surgeon. Should the bullet be removed at the time of debridement? If it lies dangerously deep in the brain, should it be left in place? Or should the surgeon perhaps extract it at a later date by means of a stereotaxic probe, which is a special probe guided to a destination deep in the brain by extremely accurate measuring devices, checked by serial x-ray films?

Experience in war surgery has shown that a bullet or shell fragment, if readily accessible, should be removed, for this lessens the chances of infection from any bacteria it might have carried. If it lies deep in the brain, however, it should be allowed to remain there, for the chances of infection are small compared with the risk of serious brain damage from hunting for it surgically. The first soldier I operated on in North Africa during World War II to this day retains the offending shell fragment deep in his brain, as I dared not search for it while cleaning up his scalp and skull wounds. Despite this, he has enjoyed a good life, with full employment.

Modern stereotaxic probing, which is not available in most hospitals and which requires unusual skill, now permits the extraction of deep-lying bullets or shell fragments without additional injury to the brain, provided they do not lie next to a vital area that might be injured by the procedure and thus cripple the patient. The only reasons for considering stereotaxic extraction are to avoid the ever-present, although slight, risk of infection from the bullet or to prevent its slow migration by gravity to a deeper and vital area of the brain, where it could produce serious symptoms like partial paralysis or even, as in one case I have seen, uncontrollable tremors.

Consideration of this gruesome topic inevitably stirs memories of a tragic assassination in the 1960s. While I do not know in detail the exact nature of the wound, it is clear that there had been a mortal bullet wound low in the back of the head, where the most important part of the brain, as far as life is concerned, is situated. This is the brainstem. It consists, as most modern high school graduates know, of the medulla—its lowermost or farthest back portion, which joins the spinal cord; the pons, from the Latin for bridge, at its center, which forms a bridge between the cerebellum or little brain and the brain and spinal cord; and the midbrain, farthest forward, which connects the brainstem with all the rest of the brain.

Injury to the medulla stops breathing, but not necessarily the heart, which may go on beating if breathing is maintained artificially. Serious injury to the pons or to the midbrain will paralyze all muscle control, and result in coma and drastic alterations of heart rate and breathing that can quickly prove fatal. Midbrain injury may also lead to abnormal eye movements and perhaps even blindness should the person recover consciousness.

From this account it is readily apparent why a gunshot wound in the back of the head is apt to be fatal. Even if the bullet does not slice the brainstem, there is usually so much bleeding that a large blood clot occurs, resulting in intense pressure that damages the brainstem beyond hope of recovery. And even if life can be saved by surgically removing the clot, there has generally been enough damage to the brainstem to cripple the victim permanently, mentally as well as physically.

If fractured bone fragments have to be removed, this will leave a hole in the skull that allows the scalp to sink in slightly. For protective and cosmetic reasons it is often advisable to repair the defect. This requires a second operation, for the surgeon must first be certain that the original wound has not become infected. Because this is cranial plastic surgery, it is called a cranioplasty. It involves reopening the scalp to insert a hard substance, such as a bone graft, a metal plate, metal mesh, or a plastic material.

Actually, the cheapest, most effective, and easiest material to use is aluminum mosquito netting! A piece of this screening is cut and molded to the desired size and shape, so that it fits neatly over the bone defect, and is coated with a fast-setting plastic substance that quickly makes it as hard as rock. It is then anchored firmly in place by delicate stainless steel wires.

Blood Clots on the Brain

One of the most common operations performed by a neurosurgeon is removal of a blood clot inside the head, formed as a result of a head injury—sometimes an apparently minor one. This type of clot, or hematoma, occurs most frequently just under the dura—which lines the inside of the skull as well as the spinal canal—and the outer surface of the brain. It is therefore named a subdural hematoma. Such clots develop when a vein on the surface of the brain is snapped by a jarring injury and bleeds. Although the bleeding may stop, these clots often become gradually larger by absorption of fluid and serum and exert more and more pressure on the brain.

Consider Mr. T., forty-two years of age, a successful, healthy broker, who was brought to our medical center by ambulance, at the request of his family physician, because for three weeks he had become progressively drowsy, suffered from headaches and failing memory, and at times either fell asleep or became completely unconscious while simply sitting in bed reading a newspaper or talking with his wife. There was no history of any past illness, high blood pressure, or known injury.

On his admission, he was so drowsy that he could not give an account of himself, his home address, or even his wife's first name. Neurological examination showed that the pupil of his left eye was larger than that of the right and that there was congestion of the optic nerve inside each eye, indicating pressure within the head.

It was clear that the trouble was on the left side of his head because pressure on that side had caused the corresponding pupil to enlarge and the opposite, or right, arm and leg to become weak and exhibit abnormal reflexes.

I explained to his wife that I did not think he was suffering from a stroke or a brain tumor. A stroke would have resulted in a more sudden reduction in his state of consciousness, while a brain tumor would more likely have caused a steady rather than an intermittent decline in consciousness. His rapid changes from practically full awareness to apparently sudden sleep were more typical of a subdural hematoma.

Mrs. T. was certain that her husband had not injured his head in any way during the last few weeks.

I asked again about a possible blow to the head, even a rather mild one, like striking the forehead against a shelf, automobile door frame, or the branch of a tree, because a subdural clot, which I suspected, can be caused by a sharp blow that quite often is not bad enough to cause unconsciousness. Thus several days or weeks may go by before the clot swells to a size sufficient to cause pressure signs. But neither Mr. T. nor Mrs. T. could recall any injury.

The next step was to proceed with x-ray and other tests, like those used for detecting brain tumors, to find out what and where the trouble was.

The tests revealed a subdural clot on the left.

At operation, the hematoma proved to be nearly an inch thick, and it was pressing down the left side of the brain. It was quite an easy matter to remove all of the clot through a small opening in the bone. When Mr. T. woke up from the anesthesia, his right-sided weakness had already cleared up, the left pupil was no longer enlarged, and even his memory had improved.

A few days later, his memory now completely normal, Mr. T. said: "Why, yes, Doctor, I *did* bang my head —it happened about six weeks ago while I was clearing brush back of the house. I turned quickly and banged my forehead against the branch of a tree. It dazed me a little for a second or so, and I thought nothing of it until now. Then headaches set in, and my mind wouldn't seem to work quite right, and—well, you know the rest."

Concussion and Contusion

Most head injuries do not cause hemorrhage or fracture but simply concussion of the brain from which recovery is usual. Concussion means a state of temporary unconsciousness caused by a sharp jarring injury to the head. As every boxer knows, when a haymaker lands on the chin, the head is jarred sharply backward. But the brain inside, like firm jelly inside a wooden box, remains stationary for a bare fraction of a second—just long enough for the inside of the rapidly moving skull to bang against the brain. In an automobile accident, when the head is flung violently forward against the dash, the reverse is true. In this instance, the swift forward motion of the skull is abruptly stopped, but the brain inside continues to travel forward. Consequently, the moving brain smacks itself against the stationary skull. The result in either case is the same: a severe jolting injury that temporarily interrupts the brain's normal electrical activity.

If the blow is mild, as from striking one's head against a shelf, the person may merely feel momentarily dazed— a mild form of concussion. A more severe blow, however, will render the person unconscious for a period of time ranging from a few seconds to several days, depending on the force of the injury. Prolonged disruptions of brain activity after a severe concussion may be caused by many tiny pinpoint brain hemorrhages as well as actual injury to some of the microscopic-sized connections between nerve cells. Repeated concussions may ultimately create so many of these tiny internal brain injuries that permanent diffuse brain damage ensues, sufficient to cause a boxer to become "punchy." This is because so many nerve cells or their connections have been damaged that the brain no longer functions normally.

A puzzling feature of severe brain concussion is that memory of events immediately preceding the blow or accident is usually lost forever. The severity of the injury determines the duration of memory loss. A friend of mine, for example, who was unconscious from brain concussion for thirty-six hours after a very bad automobile accident cannot yet remember anything of the preceding eight days. Had he been unconscious for only thirty-six minutes, his memory loss might only have been for eight hours prior to the accident.

Treatment of concussion consists of rest for one to

six weeks, depending on the severity of the injury. Otherwise the person may be subject to recurring headaches, dizziness, and weakness for two to three months. After a really severe concussion, as incurred in football or boxing, the risk of another concussion soon after should be strictly avoided because it can lead to such severe and long-lasting symptoms as just enumerated.

Contusion, or bruising, of the brain may be caused by the same type of sudden deceleration that results in concussion, but it follows a much more severe blow. The effect on the brain, usually its more forward portions, is somewhat as if a direct hammer blow to the brain had caused the local damage, characterized by oozing of blood and softening of the brain. The victim may recover perfectly, although more slowly than after a concussion. However, if vital areas such as the motor, speech, or visual cortex have been badly contused, permanent defects in motor performance, speech, and vision may ensue. A cut, or laceration, of the brain may have similar effects.

When a great deal of brain tissue has been badly bruised, as in a bad automobile accident, the congestion of the bruised parts tends to spread to other parts of the brain and make the whole brain so swollen and waterlogged that it ceases to function. The result is a prolonged state of unconsciousness, called coma, that may last for days, weeks, or—if there has been too much permanent brain damage—for years. Coma means that the person is not only unconscious but unable to speak or move his arms or legs voluntarily. There may, however, be involuntary reflex movements of the arms and legs, and staring movements of the eye (doll's eyes) that make the comatose person look as if he were awake. Coma is an ominous sign because it signifies profound brain damage from which the person may never recover. Children are more likely than adults to stage a complete recovery from coma following a head injury.

It is often difficult to know whether a person is simply unconscious or in coma. Doctors can usually distinguish between the two states because of characteristic alterations in various reflexes that they test and because the unconscious patient gradually tends to show signs of recovery, whereas the comatose patient does not.

A lad fourteen years of age whom I treated recently was badly injured in an automobile accident and was brought to the hospital in a state of coma, in which he remained for eight days. Gradually, however, he staged a complete recovery to his normal high intellectual level. Treatment consisted of bed rest and the administration of cortisone-like agents called steroids that reduce congestion of the brain. While desperately ill, he also had to be fed by vein and stomach tube. Because he had trouble breathing, a plastic tube was inserted, by an operation called a tracheotomy, into the trachea, or windpipe. If these measures had failed to improve his condition, brain surgery would have been considered to relieve the pressure in his head. This type of surgery, known as a decompressive procedure, would have entailed the removal of a large area of skull bone and probably the removal of swollen or bruised brain tissue that could be safely spared, such as that from a frontal or temporal lobe. Care was always taken at the patient's bedside to talk as if he were fully awake, for sometimes a person who seems to be in a coma may be on the verge of waking up. If he were to hear discouraging words at such a time, it might easily retard or even prevent his recovery.

Any bruise, cut, or scar of the brain may lead to epileptic fits, seizures, or convulsions. If, however, fits first occur within the first week after the head injury, they are less apt to occur again in later years. But persons having three or more fits during the first year after their injury, first occurring two or more weeks after the accident, are apt to have additional fits in the future.

Brain Surgery

In dealing with head injuries, one always comes back to the skull. For all its marvelous protective value, it is still a closed box, a fact which can prove dangerous when it contains a swollen brain under too much pressure. This is obviously why there are times when a brain surgeon must open it. It is also why brain surgery differs significantly from all other types of surgery, for the brain surgeon can never operate without considering the mechanics of pressure. And he must also know the best chemical or pharmaceutical as well as the best surgical methods for alleviating or reducing pressure.

There is an exciting new development that may someday restore sight to persons who have become blind because of a head injury that has damaged both optic nerves or, for that matter, persons who are blind for other reasons. This development involves wiring the brain so that light from the right or left, or from an up or down direction, activates the wires and tells the brain where the light is coming from. The patient is made aware of the light by experiencing a sensation of dots or lines of bright light whenever an appropriate wire or wires are activated.

The technique requires brain surgery for the application of eighty or more fine wires to the visual cortex of the brain—which is a strip of the surface gray matter in what is known as the occipital lobe, at the very back of the head. This strip is the ultimate receiving station in the brain for vision. After the wires are placed on the surface of the visual cortex, their outer ends are passed through the scalp, where they can be plugged into a photoelectric device that senses light and the outlines of objects. Photoelectric signals are then translated into electrical signals which stimulate the visual cortex, where they induce crude sensations of light. There is already an electrical device that translates printed letters into signals transmitted to the skin of a blind person, thus enabling him to read. It is hoped that technical improvements will eventually lead to a really useful degree of vision.

A similar technique is being developed with the hope of restoring hearing to deaf persons. In this case wires from a sound rather than a light detector would be applied to the brain—either at the upper margin of each temporal lobe, which is the ultimate receiving station for hearing in the brain, or perhaps to the hearing, or acoustic, nerve itself.

These developments are cited as examples of efforts that are continually under way to try to help victims of crippling brain and skull ailments, including those that lead to blindness or deafness.

4

Epilepsy

Epilepsy is about as common as diabetes, and it is estimated that there are nearly four million epileptics in the United States alone. Yet, thanks to modern methods of diagnosis and treatment, close to half this number enjoy freedom from attacks, while in another 30 percent, according to material published by The Epilepsy Foundation of America, in Washington, D.C., the frequency of seizures is minimal because of appropriate treatment. Only about 20 percent fail to respond well to medication.

Epilepsy is a term applied to an affliction characterized by spells, fits, or convulsions of various kinds, also known as seizures, to which a person is intermittently subject. The word *epilepsy* is derived from the Greek for "seizure," implying that a person is seized by something beyond his control. Some seizures are so brief and mild that they either pass unnoticed by casual observers or are thought to be a blank spell of inattention. Other seizures are so sudden and violent that a person may fall and suffer uncontrolled stiffening and then thrashing of the muscles: a convulsion. Still other varieties are characterized by uncontrolled bizarre thoughts, sensations, or behavior. Some persons experience only one type of seizure, while others may be subject to more than one variety.

"A world *Who's Who* of epilepsy would be a notable volume," Dr. William G. Lennox (1884–1960), an eminent American authority on this affliction, wrote in *Epilepsy and Related Disorders*. As he pointed out, many famous persons have been epileptics who refused to allow their occasional attacks to interfere with their pursuits. They triumphed over their disease even without the specific medicines and other methods of treatment available today.

Among those cited by Lennox and others were Amenhotep IV (Akhenaton) of Egypt; Pythagoras, Empedocles, Democritus, and Socrates of ancient Greece; Julius Caesar and Caligula of ancient Rome; Charles V of Spain; Louis XIII of France; and William Pitt, Prime Minister of England. Distinguished writers included Dante, Dickens, Molière, de Maupassant, Dostoevski, Flaubert, and Lord Byron. Paganini, Handel, and Tchaikovsky, composers, and Edward Lear and Van Gogh, artists, were others on the list, which also included Napoleon Bonaparte and Alfred Nobel. Epilepsy need not prevent or even cripple success.

The brain disorder causing epilepsy seldom leads to mental retardation and the convulsions it causes seldom lead to any physical harm. Moreover, the fact that a child or an adult has a convulsion does not necessarily mean that he is an epileptic. Infants and young children may have convulsions for reasons never explained, from which they recover perfectly without ever having another. Some may have convulsions only when they have a high fever. Convulsions may also be caused by a very low blood sugar, a brain tumor, or an angioma of the brain.

Causes

Why does epilepsy occur? What causes spells during which a person, like a marionette, is manipulated physically, emotionally, or intellectually by the nerve strings of his own brain? The answer is that something has gone wrong with the electrical activity of the brain—some of the nerve cells have become temporarily overactive or their natural rhythm has become upset. Nearly 100 years ago Hughlings Jackson, a famous British neurologist and a pioneer in the study of epilepsy, described it as a state induced by the "sudden, violent, disorderly discharge of brain cells." In simple terms, this means an electrical brain storm, or what one doctor, without meaning to be facetious, called "static in the attic."

In most kinds of epilepsy, these electrical storms arise in the surface layer, or cortex, of the brain. Immediately below the cortex lie the nerve fibers that constitute the wiring system of the brain: the white matter. Nerve cell clusters therein, which serve as relay and regulatory stations for the cortex above and the spinal cord below them, may also give rise to brain storms that cause certain kinds of seizures.

The electricity in the brain comes from the nerve cells themselves, each tiny cell being a miniature power plant that generates all the electrical current necessary for receiving and transmitting nerve signals or messages. The combined output of these tiny currents is enough, with amplification, to create the record of brain waves known as an electroencephalogram, or EEG.

Brain storms causing spells or convulsions are usually the result of some kind of brain defect, damage, or disease. A baby may be born with defective development of some part of the brain because something has gone wrong during its growth before birth or the brain may have been physically damaged during the birth process. There might be an inherited tendency to faulty brain development, or perhaps the mother had some serious disease or took a dangerous drug during pregnancy. Brain damage incurred later in life may be caused by a brain scar resulting from a head injury, infection, or poor circulation of blood. Rare degenerative, wasting diseases of the brain may also lead to seizures. In some cases the cause cannot be determined.

There are several theories as to why a brain defect or scar causes a brain storm. One possibility is that nerve cells have been irritated by a brain scar and therefore stimulated into an overactive, disorganized state. Another possibility is some drastic change in the number or quality of the signals that bombard cells rendered supersensitive by an adjacent defect or scar. Too many signals, such as those that may arise as the result of intense emotional excitement, may overexcite these sensitive cells and result in a seizure.

It is also possible that the normal system of checks and balances between nerve cells is altered in such a way that a brainstorm occurs, for every cell functions according to a dual STOP and GO system of control. A cell will discharge a signal when stimulated by signals from related cells—the GO principle. But it can be inhibited from action by receiving messages from other cells whose special function is to say: "STOP! Don't get excited and fire off any signals." If, however, these special inhibitory cells are themselves put out of action, as they are by some drugs, the cells they govern will go wild. The result can be a violent convulsion.

Another, better documented cause of seizures is a chemical change that alters the usual electrical activity of nerve cells. The chemical change may come from within the brain itself, if one of the adrenalinlike substances manufactured by nerve cells becomes either overabundant or deficient. These substances play a role in the transmission of every nerve signal. Any spontaneous or imposed drastic alteration of their amount can therefore alter the degree of activity of brain cells sufficiently to cause a brain storm.

— Chemical changes originating outside the brain may also touch off a seizure. Nerve cells are extremely sensitive to chemical changes and do not function properly if deprived of their accustomed supply of oxygen, sugar, calcium, or other nutritive substances brought to them by the blood. Hormone changes, like those during puberty, or congestion (edema) of the brain from too much fluid accumulation, may also alter the natural chemical environment of nerve cells and precipitate a seizure. Anyone having seizures of any kind should obviously be promptly and thoroughly studied in order to find the cause and institute treatment.

Common Types

The four most common types of epilepsy are: petit mal, focal seizure, generalized seizure or grand mal, and psychomotor seizure.

Petit mal, from the French for little sickness, is a seizure pattern characterized by brief episodes of apparent mental blankness during which the person seems momentarily out of contact or "day dreaming." He may acquire a blank look, appear to stare without seeing, and be unable to respond to what is said to him. During such attacks some people really do not know what is going on around them, whereas others can keep track of a conversation and follow it up once the seizure is over. Spells of this kind may be caused by a brain storm in the deep gray matter of the brain. They last five to twenty-five seconds and, in rare instances, may occur as many as one hundred times a day, generally in children from five to fifteen years old.

When these children have such lapses at school, they are often accused of not paying attention or else are considered mentally retarded because their spells have prevented them from learning all they should. Teachers, who are sometimes the first to detect such seizures, can do a lot to help such children. First of all, they should report their observations to the parents so that medical attention can be provided. Second, a teacher can be helpful psychologically by understanding the condition and thus encouraging, rather than discouraging, the pupil. Third, if other children in the class have noticed the seizures, the teacher can be extremely helpful to the epileptic child by explaining the situation to the other children so that they do not regard the child with fear or contempt but treat him like anyone else in the class.

A focal seizure or convulsion is one that begins with, and is usually limited to, trouble in just one focus (portion) of the brain. Suppose, for example, that the nerve cells that control the right index finger are triggered into abnormal activity by a local electrical storm in the brain. The index finger will then twitch uncontrollably. Sometimes the brain storm spreads to neighboring nerve cells, such as those that control other fingers, and then to cells controlling the wrist, arm, face, and leg muscles, generally in that order. This leads to a progressive spread of convulsive movements from one set of muscles to the next, called a march.

The involuntary rhythmic twitching usually becomes more and more rapid and violent and then subsides after a few final, vigorous, and irregularly timed muscle jerks. There may then be temporary weakness or paralysis of the involved muscles, presumably because the nerve cells are exhausted and unable to function for a while. The person is usually conscious during such focal attacks, and able to hear, see, understand, and talk. Sometimes, however, consciousness may temporarily be lost.

Focal seizures confined to muscular movements are called motor seizures. There are, however, other varieties of focal seizures. One of the most common is a sensory seizure, so called because the local brain storm involves nerve cells of the sensory cortex, directly behind the motor cortex. Such an attack may begin with a feeling of numbness or tingling in the index finger. This bizarre sensation may then march up the arm and then involve that entire side of the body, exactly as does the march of a motor seizure.

Difficulty with expressive speech—that is, in finding the right words, although knowing perfectly well what one wants to say—may also herald the onset of a focal seizure. In like manner, a distortion of hearing may be caused by a seizure beginning in the auditory cortex of the upper and outer portion of a temporal lobe.

Other parts of the temporal lobe, and also the cortex near the very back of the brain, are concerned with the interpretation of what is seen. A focal seizure in these areas, which are the principal and final receiving stations for vision, is apt to cause sensations of flashing lights, zigzag lines, spots before the eyes, or even well-formed visual images of scenes that may either be imaginary or have been witnessed by the person years earlier.

Less frequent kinds of focal seizures are those that begin with turning of the eyes toward the right or left. These are known as adversive seizures, from the Latin *ad* (toward) and *versive* (turning). There are two principal areas on each side of the brain in which this type of attack may be initiated. An electrical storm that activates either of these areas on the left side of the brain forces the eyes to turn toward the right, while corresponding areas on the right force the eyes toward the left.

Common to many focal seizures is the victim's awareness that something is going wrong—a type of what is known as an aura.

Another fairly common characteristic of focal seizures is that they are not necessarily confined to only one group of muscles or to disturbances of sensation alone. They may spread to adjacent nerve cells until not only muscle control and sensation in an arm are affected but also other functions such as articulation. Finally, a brain storm beginning as a focal seizure may sometimes spread across the interconnecting nerve fibers that link the two sides of the brain. Both sides of the body will then be involved by the convulsion, which is described as a generalized seizure.

Generalized seizures (also called grand mal, from the French, great sickness) may begin as a focal attack, or may occur without any warning. In the latter case, the victim cries out and slumps unconscious to the floor, whereupon the muscles of both sides of the body first stiffen and then thrash at an increasingly rapid, rhythmic tempo. There may be loss of bladder control, color changes in the face, some temporary trouble in breathing, and excessive secretions of mucus that look like foaming at the mouth. Generally these attacks are brief, so that after a few minutes, when the person comes to and rests, he can resume his usual activities.

When such an attack, or for that matter, any other seizure, recurs immediately after the first one and leads to a continuous series of seizures it is known as status epilepticus. Grand mal attacks may be the result of a brain storm arising either in the deep gray matter of the brain, or from some portion of the cortex, frequently that of one or both frontal lobes.

Psychomotor seizures are a less common form of epilepsy and may have a variety of symptoms. They are characterized partly by psychic disturbances and partly by abnormal motor activity—the latter taking the form of automatic but coordinated movements, called automatisms, as opposed to the twitching convulsive movements typical of a true motor seizure. These coordinated movements may be of various kinds. Some consist of smacking of the lips and mouth; others take the form of walking or running through city streets or across country for as much as a mile without the person's being aware of what he is doing. Still others take the form of violent assaults, sometimes with intent to kill. Rage reactions of this assaultive type are one form of psychic disturbance typical of some psychomotor seizures. Other psychic manifestations include hallucinations of various kinds, such as seeing visions, hearing imaginary music, feeling confused, or being subject to "forced thinking," which means that thoughts, often inconsequential, keep crowding into the mind.

Most such seizures are caused by malfunctioning of either the right or left temporal lobe. These lobes contain in their depths nerve relay stations that are important for the control of emotions, which explains why emotional control may be lost, leading to violent rage in some persons and serious feelings of depression in others. Abnormal activity of temporal-lobe nerve cells concerned with digestion explains why some psychomotor attacks are accompanied by smacking of the lips, or in young children, by a sensation of cramps and pain in the stomach. Most of these symptoms arise from disturbances in the deep forward portions of the temporal lobes.

Farther back, the upper portions of the temporal lobes are concerned with the integration and interpretation of visual and auditory sensations. If these areas become disturbed, visual or auditory hallucinations occur.

Two other characteristics of temporal-lobe seizures deserve mention. One is an aura that causes the victim to feel that he has already seen or experienced the scene at hand, and that, contrary to actuality, it is completely familiar. This phenomenon is known from French as déjà vu, or already seen. Another, less common aura is a sensation of a disagreeable odor, such as burning rubber. This reflects a disturbance within the innermost portion of the lobe, which is a cortical receiving station for the sense of smell.

Diagnosing Epilepsy

No one knows why seizures are not always continuous, as they are in certain rare cases. This is particularly puzzling since the EEG in most epileptic persons usually reveals some disturbance of the brain waves, called dysrhythmia, even at times when no attack is occurring. Presumably, therefore, seizures occur only when the electrical brain storm builds up to a critical pitch.

The diagnosis of epilepsy, like that of any other disease, depends on a detailed history of exactly what happened and when. Was there any family history of epilepsy? Any complications at the time of birth? Any head injury or serious infection or other symptoms of disease in the recent or remote past? Precisely what happened when seizures occurred? Did they begin with a focal seizure in just one part of the body, and if so, what part? Or did they affect all the muscles of the body at once?

Thorough examination of the patient is next in order, to see if there are any clues, based on abnormal reflexes and other findings, that might indicate what part of the brain is responsible.

Special tests, in addition to routine studies of the blood and urine, include x-rays of the skull and an electroencephalogram. Of all the tests the EEG is by far the most important preliminary one. This test can show not only what part of the brain is misbehaving but also how it is misbehaving. This information helps determine what kind of seizures the person has and how they can best be treated. (In some cases, however, the EEG fails to give an answer.)

The EEG test is a simple one for the patient. It is performed while he is lying comfortably on a table, with sixteen or more wires attached to his scalp and connected to the recording apparatus. The patient feels no pain, electrical sensation, or shock. If the EEG appears normal in persons suspected of having epilepsy, a disturbance of the electrical rhythm of the brain may often be brought to light by having the person breathe vigorously. This hyperventilation alters the blood chemistry enough, in some instances, to make faulty nerve cells misbehave and thus reveal their presence on the EEG. Another method is to have the person go to sleep or become drowsy during the test, either by encouraging sleep or by giving a mild sedative, for during sleep an abnormal EEG pattern may emerge that does not appear when the person is awake. Still other methods include stimulating the brain cells by the use of drugs or by rhythmic flashes of light.

The EEG test usually takes only thirty to fifty minutes. Contrary to what some people believe, it does not read the mind, tell a person whether he is mentally or emotionally ill, or have any curative effect.

A normal EEG, with the subject awake, is characterized by brain waves having a frequency of eight to twelve per second. Their height or "amplitude," as traced on the moving paper, indicates the amount of electrical current or "potential" of each wave in terms of microvolts (thousandths of a volt). Normally this is in the range of twenty to sixty microvolts.

The four types of epilepsy are characterized by wholly different types of brain waves. When recorded on the moving paper of EEG tests, these brain waves form four distinguishing patterns, representing the four types of epilepsy. While these characteristic EEG findings are not necessarily present in every case, 85 percent of all epileptic persons show some kind of EEG abnormality, even in seizure-free periods.

Treatment

The immediate treatment of the kind of epilepsy that results in a motor convulsion is to let the person lie on a bed, sofa, or the floor until the attack is over, and to loosen clothing that might interfere with breathing. It is not advisable to try to restrain movements except to prevent injury. The mouth should not be forced open nor anything put between the teeth, but if the mouth is already open, a handkerchief may be placed between the teeth, on one side only, to improve breathing. (Fortunately, choking is extremely rare.) The head should be turned to one side so that saliva can run out of the mouth. If seizures persist, a doctor should be called at once to give an injection of an anti-convulsant medicine. Otherwise, when the seizure is over, the person may simply swallow another tablet or capsule of whatever medicine he has been taking, to ward off another attack, and go about his usual business. (This applies to known epileptic patients who are accustomed to their attacks, and is quite a different situation from persons experiencing a convulsion for the first time, who demand prompt and thorough diagnostic efforts to discover the cause of their attack.)

The long-term treatment of epilepsy, by medicines, obviously depends on the nature and cause of the seizures. Certain of the twenty-five major anti-convulsant medicines prevent, or at least reduce the frequency of, some kinds of seizures, while others are specifically for other kinds. The specialist, usually a neurologist, knows which medicine is the best and how much of it should be prescribed. Most of the medicines act by damping the overactivity of the super-sensitive nerve cells and are not addictive. Through the National Epilepsy League, Chicago, Illinois, they can be purchased considerably below retail costs.

An interesting new approach to the treatment of epilepsy relies on computer techniques that have now been developed, which quickly analyze many different kinds of brain waves—some not even detectable by an ordinary EEG. This had led Professor José Delgado of Yale University, on the basis of experiments on monkeys, to suggest the possibility of stopping otherwise untreatable epilepsy by having a computer translate epileptic brain waves into electrical stimuli, which, when sent back to the brain, inhibit or stop these abnormal epileptic brain waves and therefore prevent convulsions.

Surgery relieves some but not all kinds of epilepsy. Psychomotor seizures, if clearly confined to one temporal lobe, respond extraordinarily well to removal of the forward part of that lobe, and the removal does not affect the brain's functions or the patient's well-being. The following case illustrates this and also shows how a person may suffer different types of seizures at different times.

Miss C., twenty-two years of age, was so depressed by having two to five epileptic seizures each day, in spite of appropriate medication, that she had attempted suicide and was therefore placed in a mental hospital. From there, in the hope that brain surgery, as a last resort, might relieve or cure her, she was transferred to our medical center.

Her epilepsy story had begun when she was nine years old, with a generalized seizure shortly after a bout of measles, mumps, and then whooping cough. Each is a virus disease, and any one could have affected the brain. When Miss C. was fourteen, the seizure pattern changed to sensations of "closing of the left ear," seeing circles out of the left corner of each eye, and numbness of the left side of the face. These were of course focal symptoms related to hearing, vision, and skin sensation, caused by a disturbance on the right side of the brain. Each attack culminated in unconsciousness and falling, followed by stiffening of the muscles, and then to-and-fro thrashing movements. Here then was an example of focal attacks that became converted by a spreading brain storm into generalized grand mal seizures.

By the time she was eighteen, the pattern changed again. There were fewer generalized convulsions. Instead, she experienced "scary feelings," a sense of "floating," or seemed to hear distant sounds. At times there were also forced ideas that interrupted the train of thought, and automatic movements. The latter consisted of smacking of the lips, posturing of the arms like poses of a ballet dancer, or forced pacing up and down the room in a trancelike state. All these manifestations were typical of temporal-lobe psychomotor seizures.

Examination of the patient showed no external signs indicating brain damage. However, EEG tests always showed a mild but definite slowing of the brain waves over the right temporal area. Other tests, customarily used to detect a brain tumor, showed nothing else wrong with the brain.

Because of her desperate plight and the fact that medicines had failed, brain surgery was recommended. The operation, performed as if for a brain tumor, was carried out under local anesthesia and moderate sedation, so that the patient would be awake. This permitted better evaluation of EEG recordings during surgery, which proved extremely useful, for they showed far more clearly than the preoperative recordings from the scalp exactly where the trouble lay: in the forward portion of the right temporal lobe. These recordings now revealed large spike-like waves, which became even more prominent and more frequent when she had a mild seizure on the operating table. This part of the temporal lobe was therefore removed.

Since surgery Miss C. has suffered no further seizures but as a precaution has continued taking the same medicine she had been given prior to the operation. In addition, she no longer feels depressed, has made a good social adjustment, and has been working full time.

Other types of epilepsy can also, although less often, be alleviated by removal of scarred or diseased portions of the cortex—provided these can be cut out without harming the patient. Such operations are sometimes helpful for another reason: they may disclose an unsuspected but easily removable tumor, cyst, or unusual blood vessel so small that it was not revealed by the usual complement of special tests. Removal generally means that seizures are stopped and the patient is cured.

While epilepsy surgery is carried out in much the same manner as an operation for a brain tumor, the brain must be carefully studied during the operation by means of electrical stimulation, to find out exactly what portion, when stimulated, is responsible for the attacks. This is done by applying a small electric current, about the equivalent of that supplied by a small flashlight battery, to the exposed surface of the brain, gently touching various areas with soft wires attached to the power source. During these trials, the response of the patient is carefully observed and the electrical activity of the brain monitored by an EEG apparatus. The tip of each recording wire is covered with a tiny ball of moist cotton to protect the brain from any harm. Because this is a recording directly from the cortex, it is called an electrocorticogram. When it shows up obviously abnormal brain waves from a given part of the brain, these usually indicate the diseased or scarred area that requires removal.

Another surgical technique that is sometimes helpful

for improving certain varieties of generalized seizures is to interrupt nerve fibers of the white matter that connect one cerebral hemisphere with the other. This can be done either by a direct surgical approach or by cutting the fibers with a radio-frequency current emanating from the tip of a special probe designed for the purpose. The latter procedure is similar to the stereotaxic operations used for the treatment of Parkinson's disease and certain kinds of pain.

In conclusion, it should be emphasized again that many persons suffering epileptic seizures can now be successfully treated by medicines or by surgery so that they can enjoy life, return to work, and even obtain life insurance. They should not, however, drive a car or other vehicle without medical permission and strict attention to state laws. Finally, it is extremely important for associates and friends to treat epileptics in such a way that they feel no stigma. For many years epilepsy was considered a "shameful" disease, and if one had an epileptic member of the family it was a matter to be hushed up. I hope this chapter has demonstrated that epilepsy is a result of defectiveness in the wiring system of the brain. Like the television set or the washing machine which breaks down once in a while, only one part need be defective to upset the function of the whole. A TV system temporarily "on the blink" is not a cause for shame; and neither is an epileptic seizure.

RIGHT ON!

5

Headache

Nearly everyone occasionally suffers a headache, for this is one of the most common afflictions of the human race. Fortunately, headaches in most people do not occur very often or last very long, and they are very seldom caused by anything of a serious nature.

Persisting headaches, however, are naturally a source of worry and deserve prompt medical attention. They may be a sign of serious brain trouble, although more often some other cause is discovered, such as sinusitis or nervous tension from worry, fatigue or frustration. A persisting headache may even be caused by something as simple as muscle spasm, as in the case of Mrs. G.

Mrs. G., a hard-working, sensible neighbor of mine, recently telephoned my office because of persisting headache across the back of her head. It had plagued her, she said, constantly for a week. Then, in almost a whisper, she said, "Do you think I have a brain tumor?" I told her that I did not think so, but that I would see her in the office the very same day.

Her story, as told at the office, immediately suggested the probable cause of her pain. She had come back from a Florida vacation and after arrival at a New York airport had stood outside, with only a light coat, in a chilly, gusty wind for an hour, while waiting for the family car. The next morning she woke up with severe aching pain across the back of her head. Aspirin and other medicines prescribed by her family doctor relieved the pain for only short periods. She had never before had such headaches and had no other symptoms, except for some stiffness down the back of the neck.

My neurological examination showed that nothing was wrong except for visible stiffness of the muscles running up her neck to the back of the head. These muscles stood out so prominently that I could see and feel them. In addition to being rigid, they were tender at several points, even to gentle pressure.

"It seems clear," I explained, "that the cold wind resulted in inflammation and then painful spasm of your neck muscles—a mild form of what we call myositis—and that you do not have a tumor or any other serious trouble. When muscles tighten up too much they can be very painful, as you know if you have ever had a cramp in your leg." I prescribed a heating pad and massage for the stiff muscles, and appropriate medicine. She went home, enormously relieved to hear my diagnosis, and by the end of a week had no more pain or muscle stiffness.

Tension Headaches

One cause of tension headaches, the kind that are felt across the back of the head, is excessive tightening of these same head and neck muscles. Presumably these headaches develop because nervous tension, in some individuals and for some unknown reason, leads to painful tensing of these muscles. Tension headaches may also be experienced over other parts of the head: across the forehead, at the temples, or all over the head. They are particularly apt to afflict exceptionally high-strung, nervous, or tense persons. Any increase of tension, as from fatigue or emotional stress, can apparently "spill over" to nerves of the head and result in headache.

Some tension headaches, and certain other kinds of headache, may be caused by drastic alterations in the size of blood vessels in or around the head. These blood vessels, like skin, muscles, and other body tissues, are provided with nerves, some of which are sensitive to pain. In some individuals, nervous tension causes scalp arteries to dilate or expand so widely that their walls, and the nerves within the walls, become painfully stretched. The dilated vessels may throb with each beat of the heart and result in a pounding kind of headache. A person suffering severe sunstroke provides an extreme example of this phenomenon: the blood vessels of the victim's forehead and temples stand out and throb visibly.

In other persons nervous tension may cause a painful contraction of head arteries. This is called spasm of the artery. What happens is that the artery's caliber is narrowed by a cramping of the little muscles that encircle the artery. Such muscles control the caliber of all arteries and thus regulate the amount of blood flowing through them. The face, for example, blushes when its arteries dilate and becomes deathly pale when they are clamped shut.

No one knows exactly why blood vessels of the scalp or the brain sometimes expand or contract to an extreme and perhaps painful degree. It is possible that nervous tension floods the nerves of the blood vessels with so many nerve signals that the muscles and thus the vessels contract. An over-expansion of blood vessels, however, may be caused by an entirely different mechanism. In this instance, their encircling muscles may relax from temporary paralysis caused by some alteration of the body chemistry. The pressure of the blood will then dilate the relaxed vessel. This theory is based on the knowledge that stress can lead to drastic changes in the chemistry of the body. It affects, for example, the production of hormones, such as adrenalin, which can influence the caliber of blood vessels. Another possible explanation of some tension headaches is that stress has overstimulated nerve-cell stations deep in the brain that are concerned with sensations of head pain.

Why are some persons subject to frequent tension headaches while others rarely have them? One obvious answer is that some people are more sensitive to pain than others, while a few are incapable of ever feeling pain. So, in one person a certain physical condition produces pain (headache), while the same condition in another does not.

Another factor to be considered is the varying sensitivity to stress exhibited by different organs of the body. In one individual, for example, stress may lead to a bleeding ulcer, in another, to palpitation of the heart, and in still another, to tension headache.

An individual's susceptibility to headache may also depend on whether the natural variations of hormones and other cyclic changes in body chemistry, like those associated with the menstrual cycle, render the pain nerves in the scalp, muscles, or blood vessels of the head supersensitive and thus lead to headache. Changes in body and brain chemistry may likewise explain the headaches associated with fever, constipation, or over-indulgence in alcohol.

Sinusitis

While nervous tension is the most common cause of headache, sinusitis is also a common cause. The sinuses that give rise to headache are bony cavities of the skull that are connected by small drainage passages to the back of the nose. When these sinuses or their passages become congested, infected, or plugged by mucus or pus, severe pain can result. If the frontal sinuses, above the eyes and nose, are affected, pain will usually be felt across the forehead. Congestion or infection of a maxillary sinus, or antrum, beneath the cheek, may result in facial pain. There are still other sinuses, the ethmoid sinuses, farther back in the base of the skull. These, when plugged or congested, can give rise to excruciating pain, usually at the very back of the head. It is often very difficult to detect an infection in these deeper and more remote sinuses either by examination or by x-rays. Consequently, a brain tumor or some other serious disease may be suspected and unnecessary tests made which prolong the suffering, sometimes for weeks. In this respect I vividly recall the case of a fine young nurse whom I was asked to see some fifteen years ago.

Miss X. was suffering from constant severe headache at the top and back of her head that had plagued her almost constantly for three months. During that time many sinus examinations were carried out and x-rays taken. Numerous other studies were made to rule out a brain tumor. Nothing, however, was detected to explain her headaches. She then began to take increasingly powerful pain-relieving drugs, until finally she was considered to be a drug addict with purely psychosomatic symptoms. Her desperation from the constant pain eventually led to a suicide attempt. It was then that a psychiatrist referred her to our medical center, with the recommendation that brain surgery (lobotomy) be considered.

After careful study, I concluded that her pain was real and had a physical cause. I further suspected that she did not have a brain tumor but was probably suffering from ethmoid sinusitis. One of our first-rank nose and throat specialists was therefore called upon. He promptly discovered and removed a single lump of pus from a deep ethmoid sinus. Her headache vanished the same day, never to return. She required no more drugs and soon returned to full-time work.

Other Causes

An infected tooth can also be a cause of headache on the same side of the head as the tooth. Pain of this sort, which has a different location from the actual source of the trouble, is known as referred pain. Referred pain over the side of the head from an infected tooth is explained by the fact that the fifth cranial nerve, which supplies the teeth, has other branches. Some of these supply the dural membrane on that side of the head. If the tooth infection bombards the receiving station for this nerve with too many pain signals, the dural branches may be activated and falsely suggest that the source of the pain is in the head rather than in the tooth.

Another and very familiar example of referred pain is an ice-cream headache. Bolt down a sizable chunk of an ice-cream cone and you will be smitten by a sudden splitting headache across your forehead. The abrupt chilling of the stomach has sent an unexpected volley of nerve signals to the brain along the vagus, or stomach nerve. These overabundant signals spill over, intensely affecting closely related cells of the fifth nerve, which supplies the forehead (as well as the rest of the face, the teeth, and the dura). The result is pain in the forehead, which seems to be the predestined site for this particular kind of referred pain.

Branches of the fifth cranial nerve are also implicated in most of the headaches that arise from such rare but serious conditions as a brain tumor, a large blood clot, pressure inside the head from hydrocephalus, or swelling of the brain after a head injury or infection. These nerve branches convey sensations from the dura, and this lining of the skull is sensitive to pain caused by drastic alterations of pressure inside the head. Headache may occur because the pressure in the head is either too low or too high. Low-pressure headache occasionally occurs after cerebrospinal fluid has been removed for diagnostic purposes by a spinal tap such as that used for a myelogram. This is called a lumbar-puncture headache. High-pressure headaches are more common. An extreme example is the kind which immediately occurs after the bursting of an aneurysm, a blood vessel blister in the head. The acute increase of pressure from hemorrhage, if severe, results in a headache described by some patients as "like being hit on the head with an ax."

Pain in the head, usually back of and around one eye, may also be caused when an aneurysm of the artery directly behind the eye socket swells. Pain-sensitive nerves in the blood-vessel wall are irritated by the stretching aneurysm and pain results. The sensitivity of the brain's arteries may also explain why high blood pressure sometimes causes a pounding headache, for the high pressure within the vessels tends to expand them and thus results in painful throbbing.

Some people are subject to headaches that come in bunches, one after the other, for a day or so, or even for longer periods. These are known as cluster headaches. While their cause is not definitely known, they may be the result of chemical changes peculiar to that individual. One substance that has been blamed is histamine, a natural chemical of the body that can influence nerve transmission and activity. Treatment, consisting of histamine control by medicines, is effective in relieving some people who suffer these headaches.

Migraine and Tic Douloureux

Two special kinds of severe head pain deserve individual attention. One is migraine headache, the other tic douloureux (from the French for painful tic).

Migraine is characterized by periodic violent headaches usually confined to just one side of the head and preceded by weird changes in vision toward the opposite side of the body. (If the headache is on the left side, vision toward the right will be altered.) Migraine, also known as megrim or the megrims, sick headache (because it sometimes leads to vomiting), and hemicrania (because it affects only one half of the head, or cranium) was described in the second century A.D. by the famous physician Galen, as well as by many others before and since his time. Visual symptoms toward the opposite side take the form of shimmering zigzag lines resembling old-time fortifications. These lines, which at the onset of an attack may be black, usually develop colors and differing shapes as vivid and changeable as those of a sparkling catherine wheel. Vision may even be partially blacked out on that side. The British neurologist S. A. Kinnier-Wilson (1887–1937) commented in his *Neurology* that the " 'visions' of the twelfth-century abbess Hildegard of Bingen are . . . clearly based on the 'fortification figures,' concentric circles, and 'falling stars' " typical of migraine attacks.

Today it is widely believed that migraine headaches

are caused, in persons predisposed to suffer them, by nervous tension, extreme fatigue, or some disorder of body metabolism. The headache appears to be associated with a painful over-expansion of blood vessels of the scalp. The visual symptoms, however, are apparently associated with excessive contraction of blood vessels: the brain arteries that supply the visual cortex.

Treatment of migraine entails avoidance of extreme fatigue and nervous tension. In addition, specific medicines are now available to prevent and relieve attacks.

Tic douloureux has other names, such as trigeminal and trifacial neuralgia. The prefix tri- refers to the fact that the trigeminal, or fifth cranial, nerve has three branches. They convey all sensations from the face. The pain may be confined to one or two branches, but all three are sometimes involved. The pains are like sudden electric shocks that come and go without warning and momentarily freeze the victim with agony. Depending on the nerve branches involved, the pains may affect the chin, the cheek, the forehead, or all three.

Relief from the stabbing pains of tic douloureux is afforded in many cases by a recently discovered medicine called Tegretol, which should be taken only under the supervision of a physician, because it may cause unpleasant side effects. Another method that may provide relief is a Novocain-alcohol nerve block. If treatment by medicine fails, there are effective surgical methods of relieving these pains. This can be done by an operation at the back of the head to cut part of the trigeminal nerve or its pain pathway in the brainstem. The trigeminal nerve—the nerve that carries pain as well as other sensations from the face to the brain—may also be partly cut by approaching it through the temple bone.

Tic douloureux is not, like tension headaches, a common affliction. But, like most of the headaches described its cause has not yet been clearly established, despite considerable research. There is, therefore, a great need for continuing investigative efforts to discover the causes of headaches and better ways of preventing and relieving them.

6

Brain Tumors

It sometimes happens that a mass of new tissue begins to grow in some part of the body and creates a swelling. Such a swelling is called a tumor. Some tumors are malignant, or cancerous, but many are benign, or noncancerous. This is as true of brain tumors as it is of those occurring elsewhere in the body.

Most benign brain tumors grow just outside the brain. Such a tumor is usually a firm round lump composed of very slowly growing noncancerous cells. It is covered by a thin envelope, or capsule, that prevents it from invading brain tissues and it causes symptoms by pressing upon the brain. The capsule of a benign tumor makes it possible for a neurosurgeon to separate and peel the tumor from the brain without injury to the brain itself. A few benign tumors contain calcium which shows up in ordinary x-rays, while a few others, instead of being solid, contain cavities or cysts that are filled with either clear, yellow, or oily fluid. A cystic tumor collapses as soon as the surgeon empties it, which quickly reduces its size and simplifies its removal. In general, surgery is the only effective treatment for benign tumors, the major exception being certain pituitary gland tumors that can be shriveled up by x-ray therapy.

Most malignant brain tumors originate and grow within the very substance of the brain. For this reason they cannot be wholly removed. Parts of them, however, can be cut out and the remainder treated by x-ray and chemical therapy. In the case of slowly growing malignant tumors, such treatment can result in the prolongation of useful life for many years. Even highly malignant tumors of the brain itself or the metastatic variety that results from a spread to the brain from a tumor in another part of the body sometimes respond surprisingly well for a worthwhile period of time.

Symptoms of any brain tumor depend on what part of the brain, or which one of its nerves, is being affected. While headache is a common symptom, usually engendered by tumors large enough to cause pressure in the head, it is by no means a universal symptom. Some tumors become symptomatic without any previous warning, as in the case of Mrs. Y.

Mrs. Y., an intelligent middle-aged housewife, began the day like any other. The alarm clock went off at six, and fifteen minutes later she was in the kitchen preparing breakfast. Suddenly her right arm felt prickly and numb and then became so weak that the frying pan clattered to the floor. By the time she reached a chair, the whole right arm was twitching up and down despite every effort to hold it with her left hand. Thoroughly frightened, she tried to call her husband but could not utter a word. In a few minutes the shaking stopped, the numbness cleared, and she was able to call for help. Her husband found her pale and crying, but now perfectly articulate, so that she was able to describe what had happened. He promptly called the family physician who agreed to see her at once.

The doctor, however, found nothing wrong except for mild weakness of the right arm. He explained to the patient and her husband that she had suffered what is known as a focal convulsive seizure—a fit confined to just one part of the body, in this case to the right arm. Such a seizure indicated some sort of temporary disturbance of the left (or opposite) motor cortex of the brain. The fact that she was temporarily unable to speak, he added, meant that the speech area of the brain, which lies close to the motor and sensation nerve cells, was also briefly out of commission.

"Does this mean I have a brain tumor?" Mrs. Y. asked quietly.

"That could be the trouble," the doctor replied, "but there are other possible causes, such as a small brain scar or a circulatory problem. Even if it is a tumor, given your age, it would most likely be a benign kind that can be cured. But now it is essential that you have a few tests, in the care of a specialist, to find exactly what the trouble is and how it can be remedied."

He thereupon referred her to our hospital where I arranged the necessary tests. They revealed a tumor close to the motor and sensory area of the left side of the brain, as the family physician had suspected. At operation it proved to be a meningioma: a perfectly benign, round, firm lump that was quite easily shelled away from the brain. Mrs. Y. recovered nicely from the operation and went home ten days later in perfect health, cured.

Benign Tumors

A meningioma, the most frequently occurring benign type of brain tumor, derives its name from its origin: cells of the three membranes that cover the brain and are collectively known as the meninges. (The suffix -oma means tumor.) Since meningiomas may arise anywhere inside the skull, the symptoms they cause depend on what part of the brain they compress, as illustrated in Mrs. Y.'s case. An astonishing characteristic of some of these tumors is the fact that they can grow to an enormous size—perhaps as large as an orange—before causing any symptoms. This is because the brain can accommodate itself for a long time to a very gradual increase of local pressure without loss of function.

Mrs. Y., incidentally, was fortunate, in the sense that the diagnosis and cure of her tumor was so promptly accomplished. In many other cases, quite a long time may elapse before the diagnosis is made and the treatment carried out. In some of these cases the patient himself may be at fault, by neglecting to visit his physician or a specialist for too long a time, while in other cases the possibility of a tumor may not occur to the doctors who first see the person, as in the two following cases.

Mr. K., fifty-six years of age, was referred to my office a little over a year after his memory had begun to falter. His wife at first attributed this change to premature aging. But when serious errors in his checking account cropped up, she insisted that he visit the family physician, who she hoped would prescribe medicine to improve her husband's memory and ability to think clearly. The doctor himself thought that Mr. K. was suffering from early hardening of brain arteries—cerebral arteriosclerosis—and ordered pills designed to improve the circulation of blood to the brain. Mr. K.'s ability to think, however, continued to fail, and in addition during the ensuing six months, he became more and more depressed as well as so forgetful that he often could not even find his way home from the local store. His melancholy became so pronounced that the doctor finally insisted on psychiatric advice.

The psychiatrist felt that Mr. K.'s depression was so

serious that it might lead to a suicidal attempt. He therefore urged admission to an institution specializing in psy-
chotherapy. Here, when Mr. K. did not respond to psychiatric efforts to relieve his depression, he was given a
series of standard electric shock treatments (EST), which
often clear up depression.

Despite ten shock treatments, Mr. K. was no better,
and now began to complain of headaches. They suggested,
for the first time, the possibility of a brain tumor. A neurologist was therefore called in. He found just enough abnormalities in Mr. K.'s reflexes and signs of pressure in his
head to suggest a brain tumor. The tumor, he explained,
probably involved one or both frontal lobes, because when
they are damaged for any reason, memory failure and
depression are common symptoms.

I was called upon next and arranged appropriate tests
that did, indeed, reveal a large tumor, almost the size of
a tennis ball, in the forward part of the skull. It was clearly
pressing on both frontal lobes of the brain, which are important for thinking, memory, and emotional reactions.

At operation the large round tumor was completely
removed, at once relieving all pressure on the brain. It
proved, as suspected from the tests, to be benign—a meningioma. Mr. K. made a splendid recovery and fully regained his ability to think and remember. His usual cheerfulness was also restored and he resumed his customary
social and business activities.

Mrs. B., a thirty-seven-year-old housewife, thought
there must be something wrong with her eyesight because
when she went bowling, the ball almost always went into
a gutter instead of down the alley as usual for her. Perhaps because she lived far out in the country where there
were no specialists, the tests of vision that could have suggested the source of her trouble were not made. She was
simply told to get new eyeglasses. Six months went by,
during which vision deteriorated, and in addition, her

menstrual cycle ceased and she lost interest in sex. Her obstetrician assured her she was not pregnant, and because he felt she was too young for the menopause, he suspected a pituitary tumor, which can lead to cessation of monthly periods. It was for this reason that I was finally asked to see her. I arranged special tests for vision and pituitary gland function, and also for x-rays of the skull. All these tests clearly indicated the presence of a large pituitary tumor.

A pituitary tumor is a growth, almost always noncancerous, of the pituitary gland. Another term for it is adenoma, meaning tumor of a gland. They occur, like an enlargement of the thyroid gland called a goiter, because the cell machinery of some of the gland's cells has run amok. The result is an overgrowth of these cells that develops into a tumor.

Pituitary adenomas grow upward, sometimes to golf ball size, out of the small cup-shaped cavity in the base of the skull called, because of its shape, the sella turcica, or Turk's saddle. The sella becomes so enlarged by the pressure of such a tumor that skull x-rays show this enlargement and thus confirm the diagnosis. When these adenomas press upward upon the Y-shaped junction of the nerves for vision, they cause loss of vision toward the outer side of each eye, as if the person were wearing blinders. The result is partial blindness. Since the pituitary is the master gland that maintains full activity of the thyroid and adrenals, as well as of the sex glands, all these glands may fail to function. The victim of a pituitary adenoma may therefore become weak from lack of energy because of impaired thyroid and adrenal gland function, and sexually uninterested or impotent because of sex gland failure.

A rare variety of these adenomas causes overactivity of the other endocrine glands as well as an overproduction of the growth-stimulating hormone made by the pituitary itself. The excessive outpouring of this hormone of the pituitary gland causes an overgrowth of the bones and other tissues of the body that makes the affected person look gigantic as a result of increase in stature, size of hands and feet, and prominence of the jaws and facial bones—in some cases, to a grotesque degree. This condition is known as acromegaly (from the Greek *akros,* extremity, and *megale,* enlargement).

Small adenomas usually shrink after x-ray treatment, with relief of visual and glandular symptoms, but large tumors that have caused an advanced degree of loss of vision generally require surgical removal.

Mrs. B. at first refused surgery, which I had advised because of the large size of her tumor and the fact that she had lost a great deal of vision in each eye. X-ray therapy, the only alternative, was therefore tried. When this failed to relieve any of her symptoms, she agreed to surgery.

I explained that there are two ways of operating on the pituitary gland, one by brain surgery and the other by an operation through the nose; that each has certain advantages as well as disadvantages; and that the choice of which method to use depends on the size and nature of the tumor and the familiarity of the surgeon with one or the other approach. The approach by brain surgery involves making a small opening in the region of the right forehead through an incision wholly or mostly concealed by the hair when it grows back after being shaved for the operation. Surgery through the nose, called trans-nasal surgery, leaves no visible external scar and enables the surgeon to reach the pituitary gland from underneath rather than from its upper surface, but requires the use of a microscope and also a television screen to show, by x-ray monitoring, exactly where the tips of the surgeon's instruments are at all times. In her case, I continued, I felt that brain rather than trans-nasal surgery was best.

At operation, the main bulk of the tumor was successfully removed and she rapidly recovered full vision. The only complication in Mrs. B.'s case was that, following surgery, as frequently happens when these tumors are very large, the remaining bit of gland did not recover its capacity to stimulate other endocrine glands. Artificial gland preparations—cortisone, thyroid extract, and sex hormones —were therefore prescribed to make up for the loss of normal pituitary activity. This is called substitution therapy.

The third, less common type of benign tumor external to the brain is one that has arisen from a nerve and is therefore called a neurinoma. The usual source inside the head is the eighth cranial nerve, concerned with hearing and balance. Since this kind of tumor crushes the hearing nerve and therefore leads to deafness and often to ringing (tinnitus) in the affected ear, it is called an acoustic neurinoma. Because part of the eighth nerve is concerned with the maintenance of balance and equilibrium, such a tumor may also lead to dizziness; to sensations of whirling and swaying like seasickness, called vertigo; or even to such poor balance that the person may walk like a drunk. An example is Miss A.

Miss A., thirty-three years of age and an accomplished pianist, noticed that she was getting deaf in the left ear. Six months went by before she finally consulted an ear specialist because she had begun to experience a ringing sound, like escaping steam, in that ear and an occasional feeling of dizziness. Hearing tests and x-rays suggested to the specialist that she probably had an acoustic neurinoma of considerable size, requiring removal by brain surgery. For this reason she was referred to my office for consultation. But she procrastinated for several weeks until finally she began to lose dexterity in the use of her left arm and to stagger while walking—symptoms of serious balance and coordination difficulties that are characteristic of these tumors as they become larger. After additional very special x-ray tests had confirmed the presence and the large size of the tumor, I operated and removed it completely. Although she remained deaf in the affected ear, because the hearing nerve had been permanently damaged by the tumor, her dexterity and coordination were fully regained and she was able to resume her career as a concert pianist.

Malignant Tumors

Benign tumors constitute about half of all brain tumors detected. The other 50 percent are branded malignant because of growth characteristics that differ from those of benign tumors. As previously mentioned, the majority of the malignant variety originate and grow within the very substance of the brain. They are composed of an overgrowth of the cells that support, nourish, and hold together the nerve cells and nerve fibers of the brain. These supporting cells are called glia cells, and for this reason the tumors to which they give rise are known as gliomas—tumors of the glia. They cause trouble because, like thick vines that choke a tree, they strangle nerve cells and their connections within the brain. Fortunately, about half of all gliomas are only mildly malignant. The mildly malignant gliomas grow very, very slowly and so do not strangle or destroy nerve elements as rapidly or as extensively as do their more highly malignant cousins. A person having such a slow-growing tumor may therefore live for a long time, often without serious symptoms, providing pressure resulting from the volume of the tumor is relieved by brain surgery. In some cases this type of tumor can be totally removed, with a lasting cure; those for which this is most probable are the gliomas in children that arise in the cerebellum.

In most cases, however, the entire substance of the tumor cannot be removed without also removing invaded parts of the brain, an act that would cripple the patient. The part of the tumor that remains, however, can be treated with x-ray (cobalt) therapy and in some cases by chemical agents (chemotherapy) to slow or arrest further growth. With these methods of treatment, many persons with a mildly malignant glioma can be granted an enjoyable life for a long time, often for ten years, and in some cases even for forty or more.

Young J., a boy sixteen years old, is an example of how a mildly malignant tumor can be successfully treated by surgery and then x-ray therapy. According to his parents, he had been doing poorly in high school for about six months. His grades had dropped, apparently because he paid less and less attention in classes and neglected his homework. Like some young men of that age, he was extremely reticent in discussing his school work with his parents, saying only, "I just don't feel like working so hard."

One of his teachers, noting that he often seemed not to hear a question, urged him to see the school doctor to find out if he had any hearing difficulty. But the boy refused to do so.

A few weeks later he was dropped from the basketball team because his shooting was off. He also seemed to lose his balance and stumble at times on a fast run down the court.

By this time his parents had also noticed that his balance had become very poor and that in addition he had begun to hold his head in his hands "because of headaches." They promptly arranged a consultation with a neurologist who found that coordination and balance in the left arm and leg were badly impaired and that when J. gazed to the left, his eyes quivered from side to side with rapid jerking motions—clear signs of trouble in the left side of the cerebellum, which is concerned with balance and coordinated muscle movements. (A cerebellar, unlike a cerebral, hemisphere controls the same side of the body, not the opposite side.) In addition there was marked congestion of his optic nerves, a sign reflecting high pressure inside the head.

I was called upon to arrange tests for the suspected tumor. They confirmed its presence and location, and clearly indicated the need for surgical removal.

Operation disclosed a large fluid-filled cyst in the left side of the cerebellum. The cyst was caused by an accumulation of fluid whose source was a little nubbin or nodule of tumor about the size of a cherry. On microscopic study of a small sample (called a biopsy), the tumor proved to be a mildly malignant glioma. The cyst fluid, together with its sac or capsule, and all of the tumor nodule were completely removed.

Following surgery, young J. was relieved of his pressure headaches and gradually began to regain his balance. Cobalt therapy was given after the operation, as it is for most glial tumors, with the aim of killing any tumor remnants that might have been missed.

A year later the boy resumed play on his basketball team and did well at his studies. Twenty-four years have now elapsed with no signs of any further symptoms.

The worst kind of brain tumor, obviously, is the highly malignant variety that grows so rapidly and responds so poorly to surgical or any other type of treatment that life can seldom be prolonged for more than a few months. This kind of tumor can almost never be completely removed or destroyed and therefore keeps on growing, destroying nerve cells and their connections until the brain can no longer function properly. The mind then ceases to think, emotional control is lost, and paralysis or other symptoms, perhaps even blindness, sets in. A minor blessing at this stage is that the size of the tumor may create so much pressure in the head that the patient becomes drowsy and stuporous and does not suffer.

If all tests indicate that the tumor is highly malignant

and has already destroyed an especially important part
of the brain, like the speech area, there is no point of sub-
jecting the patient to major brain surgery. If there is any
possibility at all of there being a benign instead of a
malignant tumor, however, it is then advisable, I believe,
to perform a very small operation, through a small opening
about the size of a nickel—and under simple local anesthesia only—in order to verify with certainty the nature of
the tumor. This is accomplished by taking a small sample
of tissue which is then immediately studied under the
microscope by an expert in this art, called a pathologist.
The picture is not necessarily one of complete gloom, for
occasionally a combination of surgery, to relieve pressure,
followed by x-ray and chemotherapy, to slow tumor
growth, will restore a person with a highly malignant tumor to useful life for two or more years.

The same methods of treatment and a similar life ex-
pectancy for the patient apply to brain tumors that have
originated from the spread of a body cancer to the brain
by way of the circulating blood—a metastatic tumor—
provided that only one such tumor is growing in the brain,
and not several.

Determining the Presence of a Tumor

Three steps are required for a specialist in neurology or
neurosurgery to make the diagnosis of a brain tumor. First,
he must obtain a detailed account of every symptom and
the sequence in which it occurred. In addition, he must
ferret out any symptoms that the patient may have for-
gotten or overlooked. This is done by systematic questions
about the functioning of each of the twelve cranial nerves.
Questions are also asked concerning muscle power, balance, sensation, control of the bladder and bowels, and
whether headaches have occurred. The precise nature of

any symptom must then be determined. What was the headache like? For example, was it a tight feeling or a sensation of pulselike beating; what part of the head did it affect; and was it associated with tension, bending down, or anything else? This questioning is called "taking the history." It is an important source of information, for it alone can often tell the experienced specialist whether or not a brain tumor is the cause of symptoms. If it is, the same information can tell him the location of the tumor and its probable nature. Some of the case reports that have been cited illustrate why this is so.

The second diagnostic step is a neurological examination, meaning a systematic check of the nervous system by a series of quite simple but extremely important tests. It begins with an evaluation of how the brain as a whole is functioning. Is the person fully alert, or is he slow to understand and to respond rationally? Does he answer in a silly irrelevant fashion or cover up a faulty memory with false answers (confabulation)? These are common signs of frontal lobe trouble.

The manner of talking and walking are next evaluated, for defective performance in these functions can pinpoint the exact part of the brain that is affected. For example, an inability to name objects or express an idea, even though the patient is able to speak, indicates that something is wrong with an area of the brain dealing with speech control (on the left side of the brain in right-handed persons).

The first symptom of a tumor in a talented man of forty-five I recently saw was garbled speech. He understood perfectly everything that was said to him and clearly indicated that he knew exactly what he wanted to say but was simply unable to say it (a form of what is known as aphasia). An actual sample of his speech was as follows: "There are bottles on the apoon—dramascobular bottles [pointing to his dressing table]—uttering not nicely, you know, I am—and it hurts top-up [indicating the top of his head]." Following x-ray treatment, all these symptoms completely disappeared and he is now back at work.

The mere act of walking can supply a clue as to which side of the brain is affected, as indicated, for example, simply by how the arms swing. If one arm does not swing naturally or one leg limps, this may mean trouble on the opposite side of the brain. Poor balance, tested by the patient's standing with eyes shut and indicated by a tendency to sway or fall to one side, suggests trouble with the inner ear, with its nerves dealing with balance and equilibrium, or with the cerebellum. Cerebellar disease may also be indicated by poor coordination, as in the faulty performance of rapid or dextrous finger movements or in failure to touch accurately the tip of the nose with the index finger when the eyes are closed.

The power of arm and leg muscles is tested by comparing their degree of pull. Then the reflexes of the arms and legs are checked by tapping tendons of the arms and legs with a rubber hammer to see if the appropriate muscles jerk. Overactive reflexes on one side of the body point to trouble on the opposite side of the brain or in the spinal cord, while underactive reflexes may be caused by cerebellar disease on the same side.

Body sensations of various kinds must also be tested, for different sets or tracts of nerve fibers in the brain and spinal cord carry different kinds of sensory messages: some for pain, tested by gentle pinpricks; others for temperature, tested by touching the skin with warm or cool objects; and still others, which report the position of the limbs, joints and muscles, tested by having the person shut his eyes and then attempt to describe the direction in which his toe or finger is being moved. Another set of nerve fibers carries messages from the bones when a vibrating tuning fork is applied. There are still other tests, such as tracing numbers on the skin with a small stick of wood, to see if a person, with eyes shut, can recognize the figures. If he can feel the touch but not recognize the figures, this usually means trouble in the uppermost part of the brain's gray matter, the cortex of the parietal lobe, which is concerned with the interpretation of sensation.

The twelve nerves on each side of the brain are checked. Nerve I, the sense of smell, is tested by having the patient sniff various nonaromatic odors with each nostril. There are several tests for vision, nerve II. Is vision in each eye as sharp as it should be for the age of the person? Is the patient's ability to distinguish colors poor? This is one early sign of trouble affecting a nerve for vision. Can he see well, when each eye is separately tested, toward the right, left, up and down, or straight ahead? A defect in any one of these directions alone can tell the specialist whether the trouble is in the eye, in the nerve for vision, or in the brain itself. The interior of each eye must also be inspected with an instrument called an ophthalmoscope to see whether the optic nerve at the back of the eyeball—the only nerve of the body that can actually be seen without surgical exposure—is extraordinarily pale (which may indicate pressure on that nerve by a tumor) or whether it looks congested (a condition called papilledema) in a manner suggesting pressure within the head that may be caused by a tumor.

Other eye tests include checking whether the pupils are equal in size and react normally to light and close vision, and whether the eyeball moves up, down, or toward the nose—functions of the third cranial nerve. If an eyeball fails to move outward, away from the nose, this means that the sixth nerve is paralyzed—a sign of pressure upon it or of damage to its cells of origin in the brainstem. Fine rapid jiggly movements of both eyes (nystagmus) are caused by trouble in the cerebellum, brainstem, or eighth nerve.

Because the specialist knows the location and course

of every cranial nerve as well as a vessel's pilot knows the rocks and reefs of his home port, it is possible to chart or locate the precise site of a brain tumor as indicated by faulty action of one or more of the cranial nerves.

The sensation of the skin of each side of the face, and of the cornea or outer covering of the lens of each eye, is served by the fifth nerve on the right or left side. It is tested by gentle pinpricks of the facial skin and with a wisp of cotton for corneal sensation that should make the eye blink. The fifth nerve also controls the muscles that move the jaw which lie deep in each cheek and over each temple and must also be tested. A different nerve, the seventh, makes the muscles of the face move in facial expressions and grimaces. If all these muscles, including those of the forehead that make one frown, fail to work on one side of the face, the neurosurgeon knows that the seventh, or facial, nerve is not working. But if the forehead can be moved while the rest of the face on that side is paralyzed, this indicates that the trouble is in the brain itself—a peculiarity of the nerve supply for the face muscles. Taste must also be tested, for each seventh nerve supplies taste sensation to the forward part of the tongue on that side.

If impaired balance and rapid to-and-fro jerking of the eyes on looking to one side or the other are found, this suggests involvement of part of the eighth nerve, or possibly the cerebellum. Additional special tests are required to determine whether this nerve or the cerebellum is the cause of the trouble. Impaired hearing in one ear, which may be crudely tested by a tuning fork or a watch tick, may indicate trouble with the hearing portion of the eighth nerve. More elaborate tests for hearing are required to determine whether the deafness is really due to nerve damage by a tumor or to some other cause.

Examination of the throat muscles at the back of the mouth (ninth and tenth nerves) shows whether they move properly when the person says "Ah" and when the back of the throat is touched with a wooden applicator, causing momentary gagging. The ninth nerve also serves taste sensation for the back of the tongue. The eleventh nerve is checked by testing the strength of the muscles that shrug the shoulders and turn the head to one side, while the twelfth, which moves the corresponding side of the tongue, is tested by observing how well the tongue can be moved and whether one half of it looks withered (from paralysis). All these tests are essential, for sometimes a person himself may not be aware of trouble, especially if it has developed insidiously.

The third and final step in diagnosis includes the tests known collectively as laboratory tests. In addition to examination of the blood and urine, they include x-rays of the skull, an electroencephalogram (EEG), a brain scan, and usually other tests.

Skull x-rays do not show a tumor unless it contains calcium deposits, which a few do. But the x-rays often supply indirect evidence of a brain tumor. They may reveal a thickening of some part of the skull bone characteristic of certain meningiomas; enlargement of the sella turcica, indicating a pituitary tumor; or enlargement of the ear nerve bone channel or canal, indicating an eighth-nerve tumor. Enlarged blood vessel channels in the bone are sometimes another sign of a meningioma, while irregular thinning of the skull bone, giving it a hammered silver appearance, indicates highly increased pressure in the head that may be caused by a tumor. The pineal gland, situated nearly in the middle of the head, often contains enough calcium to show up in x-rays. If its calcium shadow is shifted, this can be another clue suggesting a tumor. Sinusitis, and erosion of bone by an infection or certain benign and malignant tumors, are also revealed by x-rays.

An EEG test, like that used for the diagnosis of epilepsy, may disclose an abnormal pattern of the brain waves that indicate the location and nature of the trouble.

Another simple, painless test is an echo-encephalogram. This is like a radar screening of the brain's fluid-containing cavities, called the ventricles. Ultrasonic waves are beamed into one side of the head and picked up by a sensitive detector on the opposite side. In a matter of minutes the detector indicates, by an electronic screen and instantaneous photographs, whether the ventricles are too large or too small, or whether they have been shifted, perhaps by a tumor, from one side toward the other.

Still another test is a brain scan. For this, a safe and tiny dose of radioactive material is injected by a small hypodermic needle. Later the entire head is scanned by the equivalent of a Geiger counter connected to a highly sophisticated computer. It rapidly prints out on paper the density of radioactivity in all parts of the brain. There is usually a high uptake of the radioactive substance at the location of a tumor.

If vision has been affected, special tests should be carried out by an eye specialist to chart the precise extent of visual loss and to determine, by other delicate tests, whether there is any disturbance of eye movements that cannot be detected by simple office examination. Similarly, if hearing or balance is impaired, the ear specialist can help pinpoint the location of trouble by a battery of sophisticated hearing tests (audiometry) and by caloric tests, meaning running cool or warm water into the ear to see if it makes the person briefly dizzy, as it normally should.

To clinch the diagnosis, for I would not operate for a brain tumor unless absolutely certain of its presence and location, I insist on either an air study or an arteriogram, and occasionally both.

An air study means that air is used to replace some of the cerebrospinal fluid in order to outline the surface and interior of the brain. Since most tumors do not show up on x-rays, and since air appears on x-rays as a "contrast" shadow, it can be used to indicate the presence of a tumor. Sometimes it literally outlines the tumor, but more often it simply shows up a displacement of a ventricle that indicates where the tumor must be. The air may be introduced by a lumbar tap like that used for a myelogram in searching for a slipped disc, or by making a small opening in the skull. A major disadvantage of an air study is that, unlike an arteriogram, it usually leads to distressing headache for a while.

An arteriogram, a visualization of the arteries also used for stroke studies, need not be uncomfortable at the time it is performed if the patient is adequately sedated. It is generally more valuable diagnostically than an air test, since it can reveal not only the location of a tumor if one is present, but also its blood supply. The latter is important for the surgeon to know about before an operation. The test may even reveal the kind of tumor. I always explain that there is a very slight risk that this test could result in a bad reaction, such as weakness or even paralysis of an arm or leg, impaired speech, or possibily a convulsion, but that the chances of any ill effects, particularly in a healthy person, are less than 1 percent, indeed so small that the value of the test far outweighs the really negligible risks.

Brain-Tumor Surgery

All the information collected from the history, neurological examination, and laboratory tests makes it possible for the neurosurgeon to know exactly where to operate for a brain tumor and what kind of tumor he may find. How is brain surgery actually performed?

In preparation for the operation, the patient's head must be shaved. After he is put to sleep by the anesthesiologist, the scalp is thoroughly scrubbed and cleansed with an antiseptic solution. Sterile towels and sheets are arranged to cover the patient except at the operative site. The scalp is then opened by a horseshoe-shaped incision that forms what is technically known as a scalp flap. Bleeding is prevented by applying clamps along the cut edges of the scalp. The flap is then lifted up and turned down and out, as if on a hinge. This exposes the bone of the skull.

Several round openings, each the size of a nickel and about three inches apart, are then made in the bone, close to the scalp edges, with a drill having a protective device that guarantees it will stop before it can possibly touch the brain. A small wirelike bone saw is then used to connect the drill holes. This creates a section of loose bone about the size of one's palm, called a bone flap, that can be lifted off the bluish dural membrane. This membrane is next carefully incised around three edges of the exposure and laid back out of the way as a dural flap. The surface of the brain is now visible. The entire procedure is called a craniotomy.

If a benign brain tumor is present, as in the cases of Mrs. Y. and Mr. K., it can be gently peeled away from the brain and removed. If it is a malignant tumor, as much of it may be removed as is possible without crippling the patient—and occasionally all of it.

Bleeding is prevented throughout the operation by lightly charring with the points of an electrocautery any small blood vessels of the brain that have to be cut. Another standard method of sealing blood vessels of the brain is to shut them off with small nonirritating metal clips.

The operation is completed by replacing all the layers of tissue just as they were. This means stitching the edges of the dura together in watertight fashion so that cerebrospinal fluid cannot leak out. The flap of bone is then snugly seated back where it was and held firmly in place either by a few delicate stainless-steel wires or by sewing together the muscles and other tissues that cover the bone. Each of the nickel-sized drill holes is usually covered with a small piece of fine innocuous metal mesh that is coated with a fast setting plastic material after shaping it to the natural contour of the skull. Finally, the scalp flap is replaced in its original position and neatly stitched. After healing, the resulting scar eventually becomes practically invisible while the shape of the head remains the same as ever.

Following the operation, the patient is moved immediately to a large wardlike room called an intensive care unit (ICU) for care by especially well-trained nurses for a day or so. The ICU has proved extremely valuable in keeping patients comfortable and guarding against any untoward complications. Although an ICU has distinct advantages as to the well-being of the patient, it has the disadvantage of being a public ward, subject to the sounds of monitoring devices and the presence of other patients.

In summary, brain-tumor surgery, while far from a pleasant affair, saves many lives and restores many persons to useful, productive, and enjoyable careers. Moreover, research with respect to the cure of malignant brain tumors is being actively pursued in this and other countries and already promises hope for the future through slowly improving methods of chemical treatment, increasing knowledge of how the principles of immune reactions may be used to halt the growth of these tumors, and perhaps the use of laser beams to destroy such tumors without the necessity of major brain surgery.

7

Strokes,
Aneurysms,
and Angiomas

During the past quarter-century, advances in the diagnosis and treatment of strokes have made it possible to cure many persons, young as well as elderly—and even young women during pregnancy—who not so long ago would have been permanently crippled or perhaps would have died.

What is a stroke? Technically it is a cerebro-vascular accident (CVA)—cerebro referring to brain and vascular to blood vessel. The term covers brain damage from the blockage of a brain artery or from hemorrhage when such an artery bursts. These are the two main causes of strokes.

Strokes Caused by Blockage

In some persons disease in an artery of the neck that supplies the brain may cause a stroke, as in the case of Mr. S., who was cured by a relatively simple operation.

Mr. S., aged sixty, president of a successful automobile agency, was watching television one night. He suddenly turned to his wife and said quietly. "Something has happened to my left arm—it's gone completely numb and I can't move it. I guess I've had some kind of stroke."

By the time the doctor arrived, about fifteen minutes later, he found that Mr. S.'s left arm now felt completely normal and was just as strong as the right. The blood pressure, pulse, and other body functions also seemed perfectly normal.

"I frankly think, Mr. S." the doctor said, "as you yourself suspected, that you have suffered a very small stroke, caused by brief interference with the circulation on the right side of the brain—the part that controls your left arm. Have you ever had anything like this before?"

"Yes—my left arm *has* felt a little funny and weak two or three times in the past month, but it cleared up so quickly I thought it was simply a touch of arthritis."

"The fact that you've had several little attacks of this sort suggests a condition that can usually be cured by a rather simple and safe operation. But you should go to the hospital in the morning for tests to see if I am right. Meanwhile, I'll give you medicine to see you through the night."

Tests at the hospital the next day showed no evidence of a brain tumor, which could have been the cause of the symptoms, whereas three special tests clearly indicated that the trouble was poor circulation through the carotid artery on the right side of the neck, the main pipeline to the right half of the brain.

The first of these three special tests was a thermogram, a simple procedure for measuring the temperature of the forehead by reflected infrared light. If a carotid artery in the neck is badly plugged, as it proved to be in this case, the forehead on that side will be cooler than the other because of a poorer blood supply.

The second test was to record, with the aid of a highly

sensitive amplifier, the sound of blood rushing through the vessel. The speed of blood flow in a narrowed (stenotic) artery is different from that in a normal one and therefore produces a different sound, typical of the condition. A familiar example of this phenomenon, an alteration of sound by speed, is the ever-lessening sound of a train's whistle as the train speeds along through the night.

The third and most crucial test was an arteriogram: a visualization of the arteries that carry blood through the neck to the brain, as well as of the brain arteries themselves. This involves the injection, under appropriate sedation or anesthesia, of a harmless liquid into a suitable artery. The liquid shows up on x-ray films and outlines blood vessels as it courses through them. In this way it can reveal anything wrong with the circulation to the brain. In Mr. S.'s case, the only sign of trouble was a pronounced thickening inside the right carotid artery, which made the artery look as if a string were tied about it so tightly that scarcely any blood flowed through. In addition, there appeared to be a small craterlike ulcer within the artery at the point of thickening. The ulcer, resembling a miniature stomach ulcer, was caused by the same kind of arteriosclerosis that caused the thickening and was the principal reason for Mr. S.'s little strokes.

In blood-vessel ulcers of this kind, small blood clots tend to form inside the ulcer. Tiny fragments can fly off the clots from time to time and be carried up into a brain artery. If they plug the artery, the blood supply is reduced —a condition called ischemia. When deprived of blood, the nerve cells supplied by a brain artery fail to function. The result is numbness, weakness, or other symptoms of brain disorder. Strokes of this kind are temporary if the tiny corklike plug, technically called an embolus, quickly dissolves or is swept away by the pressure of blood behind it. Otherwise permanent disability may ensue. The temporary strokes are called transitory ischemic attacks.

The reason Mr. S. was not permanently paralyzed, even though his right carotid artery was badly occluded, is that in most persons nature has provided an ingenious safety device. In terms of plumbing, this may be likened to pipes connected together in a circle at the base of the brain, just inside the skull. From this circle of arteries arise most of the other arteries that supply blood to the two cerebral hemispheres. The circle derives its blood supply from four major arteries that enter its under surface. These are the two carotid arteries, in the front of the neck, on either side of the windpipe, and the two vertebral arteries at the back of the neck, close to the vertebrae. The circular arrangement of vessels at the base of the brain is called "the circle of Willis," after Thomas Willis (1621–1675), a British physician famous for his studies of the circulation of blood in the brain, who described it in 1660. (The original diagram illustrating this circle was drawn for Willis by Sir Christopher Wren, later the architect for St. Paul's Cathedral.)

If one of the four main arteries is shut off by disease, the other three arteries supplying the circle tend to enlarge and to carry enough blood to preserve an adequate circulation to the brain. This is what happened in Mr. S.'s case. Blood from the opposite, normal carotid artery and the two vertebral arteries found its way through the circle of Willis in sufficient quantity to keep the brain cells on his right side alive. Willis himself pointed out this safety factor. If the circle itself became plugged, however, most of the brain cells would be so deprived of blood that they would die. Brain cells need a lot of blood—nearly a quart of blood (12 percent of all blood pumped by the heart) must flow through the brain every minute to meet the brain's requirements. In addition, the brain uses 20 percent of all body oxygen and 80 percent of all sugar made by the liver.

Mr. S.'s problem clearly called for surgical correction

of the defect in his neck artery, not only to restore it to a normal caliber but also to remove the dangerous little ulcer within it.

The operation, compared with most of those performed by neurosurgeons, is fairly simple. It requires an incision in the neck to expose the defective carotid artery. The vessel must be shut off immediately below and above the point of obstruction with special clamps. Otherwise there would obviously be a fountain of blood when the artery was opened. Before these clamps are applied, blood can be detoured around the site of the proposed repair by a temporary by-pass. A large-bore needle, aimed toward the heart, is inserted into the lower end of the artery below the portion to be clamped, while a second needle aimed toward the brain, is inserted above the obstruction. The two needles are connected by a tube so that blood keeps flowing to the brain when the clamps are applied.

The wall of the artery is then slit open and the thickened lining, along with its ulcer, is shelled out, much as one scoops out a melon while leaving its rind intact. The slit in the arterial wall is stitched closed. When the clamps and by-pass are removed, the repaired segment of the artery swells to a normal size and pulsates, as it should, with every beat of the heart.

Four weeks after the operation, Mr. S. resumed a full schedule of business and social activity and five years later has experienced no further symptoms of any kind.

Some people, not as fortunate as Mr. S., suffer more severe types of stroke caused by permanent blockage of a small but important brain artery from arteriosclerotic thickening or a clot that has plugged it. Today, however, even these conditions can sometimes be corrected by what is known as microsurgery, meaning the use of a powerful binocular microscope through which the surgeon looks as he operates.

Microsurgery

Just as scuba diving and snorkling have revealed the magic of undersea life, so has the binocular microscope, now widely used during particularly delicate neurosurgical operations, opened up new vistas of brain and spinal cord surgery, making possible operations that were scarcely dreamed of only ten years ago.

By peering through the microscope, as if through field glasses, the surgeon can see, magnified six to twenty-six times and brilliantly illuminated, tiny blood vessels, nerves, and other structures too small—or too close to vital portions of the nervous system—to be operated upon safely or effectively without magnification. A threadlike blocked brain artery looks like a shiny tube the size of one's finger. The magnification enables it to be repaired, or perhaps connected to another equally small artery, to restore circulation to a deprived part of the brain and thus relieve symptoms of a stroke. Even delicate nerves around the brain arteries, which help control their caliber, can thus be visualized during an operation. In addition, abnormally swollen veins and arteries that compress and paralyze the spinal cord, and certain rare tumors inside the very substance of the cord, can, with the aid of the microscope, be safely peeled away to restore power to weakened arms and legs. And tiny nerves, such as those of an injured finger, can be sewn together again. Microsurgery is also useful for operations on brain aneurysms and tumors close to important nerves at the base of the brain and for removing the pituitary gland to relieve pain caused by some kinds of cancer.

With such a microscope, a plugged or diseased artery can be slit open to remove an internal obstruction and then stitched together again. The stitches used are so delicate that they can barely be seen by the unaided eye. Sometimes a patch taken from the wall of an unimportant scalp vein must be incorporated in the repair to give the artery an even larger diameter than it originally had. Blood can then flow freely to the deprived area of brain and, the surgeon hopes, restore nerve cell function.

Another way of supplying blood to the brain is to connect an artery in the neck with an artery of the brain by means of a vein graft. Again the microscope must be used, not only because of the small size of the vessels but also because the slightest inaccuracy in placing a stitch can cause clotting of the repaired vessel and spoil the whole operation. Without the microscope the necessary perfection and accuracy is not possible.

Brain Hemorrhage

Bleeding, or hemorrhage, into the brain is another major cause of strokes. This usually occurs because the wall of a brain artery has become so weakened by disease—usually a variety of arteriosclerosis which softens rather than hardens a vessel—that the artery bursts and leaks blood. If the blood pressure is high, a defective blood vessel is obviously all the more apt to burst. The result, when hemorrhage is severe, is actual hydraulic destruction of brain tissue when blood squirts into it, just as water from a fire hose destroys a sandbank. If the leak is small, because of a tiny rather than a large opening in the artery and quick clotting that stops further hemorrhage, there may be little or no brain damage. However, leakage of even a small amount of blood is apt to cause headache, aching and stiffness of the neck, and sensitivity to or fear of bright light (photophobia). These symptoms are the result of the irritating effect of escaped blood when it mixes with the CSF, as it usually does, and is carried to the pain-sensitive dural lining of the brain, causing headache, and down the spinal canal, causing neck ache and reflex muscle spasm or stiffness. Irritation of the optic nerve explains the photophobia.

When a stroke has been caused by a considerable amount of blood that has squirted out into the brain, a jellylike clot called a hematoma generally results. If it is not too large and is detected promptly, such a clot can often be surgically removed with a resulting cure. An example of such a case is the following.

Mr. F., a forty-six-year-old executive known to have high blood pressure, suddenly suffered an excruciatingly severe headache, and toppled from his desk chair to the floor. His secretary found him there, moaning, holding his head in his hands, and mumbling incoherently.

Mr. F. was rushed to the hospital where the neurosurgeon, who examined him at once, found that his neck was so stiff that the head could not be moved forward, that Mr. F. kept his eyes tightly shut as if to avoid light, and that by this time he was unable to speak or to move his right arm and leg. This rapid train of events in a person with high blood pressure strongly suggested that he had suffered a stroke caused by a serious hemorrhage in the left side of his brain.

Appropriate tests were promptly arranged. The first was a spinal tap to determine whether or not there had actually been any bleeding inside the head. If so, blood usually becomes mixed with the CSF and is thus carried all the way down the spinal canal around the entire spinal cord and its nerves, where it can be easily and safely detected by a spinal tap low in the back like that used for a myelogram when a doctor is looking for a herniated disc. The spinal tap revealed blood-tinged CSF and also evidence of high pressure. It was clear therefore that bleeding had occurred, while the high CSF pressure indicated that it had probably led to a sizable hematoma causing pressure on or in the brain. The diagnosis was confirmed by an arteriogram, which revealed evidence of a large hemorrhage in the left frontal lobe.

In brain surgery directly after the test, a large blood clot was indeed found, by making a small incision through the surface of the brain at a point where the surgeon knew this could be safely done without risk of paralysis or any other serious effect. It was also apparent that this large clot had been pressing against, without actually damaging, adjacent parts of the brain dealing with speech and muscle control, which explained why Mr. F. was unable to speak or to move his right arm and leg. The clot was quickly and easily removed, almost as easily as scooping jelly from a jar, and its removal immediately relieved all pressure on the brain. The wound was then stitched up in the usual manner.

Following surgery, Mr. F. gradually regained the ability to speak and the power in his paralyzed arm and leg. At the end of three weeks he was able to go home. Now, fifteen years later, he remains well and active in business. During these years his blood pressure has been maintained at safe levels by appropriate medical treatment.

Two other causes of brain hemorrhage may also cause a stroke. One is leakage from a berry-shaped blister, or bulging, of a brain artery, called an aneurysm; the other is bleeding from a cluster of abnormal blood vessels of the brain, called an angioma.

While an aneurysm is occasionally fully formed at birth, most of them develop gradually over a period of years from a weak spot in an artery. The weak spot may be present from birth or may be caused much later in life by the kind of arteriosclerosis that softens and weakens an artery. The constant pressure of the blood within arteries causes such weak spots to bulge more and more until finally an aneurysm is formed. If the blister gets too thin and stretched, like a child's balloon blown up too hard, it may give way and either leak blood or actually burst. When this happens, the aneurysm is said to have ruptured.

Fortunately brain aneurysms are rare, with an incidence of only about 2 percent in the population at large. Less than half of all aneurysms ever bleed, but when they do bleed, they can cause symptoms resembling those of a stroke. However, some aneurysms that never bleed may become so large that they cause other symptoms, such as loss of vision or double vision from pressure upon nerves of vision or those that move the eyeballs.

The second of these two possible causes of hemorrhage, an angioma, is even less frequent and less apt to bleed than an aneurysm. The arteries and veins of an angioma are characteristically intertwined, serpentine, and usually much larger than normal blood vessels. Because they represent defective development of arteries and veins, arteriovenous malformation (AVM) is a term used to refer to this kind of angioma. The abnormal vessels generally appear on the surface of the brain, but also extend for an inch or so inside it. Some angiomas, however, lie completely buried deep inside the brain. While all angiomas and some aneurysms are present from birth, this does not necessarily mean that they are inherited or that future generations of the family will be similarly afflicted.

An angioma, as time goes on, may gradually extend over a wider and wider area of the brain and cause symptoms of brain damage, either from the pressure of its huge vessels upon the brain or because the vessels carry off blood that should feed adjacent parts of the brain. A stroke may occur when a blood vessel in an angioma becomes so thin that it leaks enough blood to form a clot. Paralysis or other symptoms then develop because of pressure or disruption effects of the clot. If leakage from an angioma or an aneurysm has been a trickle of blood that has been quickly sealed off by prompt clotting, there may be no immediate paralysis or other symptoms to suggest a stroke —only headache, stiffness of the neck, and photophobia. A few days later, however, the escaped blood may irritate adjacent brain arteries sufficiently to make them contract or go into spasm. This can reduce their caliber enough to shut down blood supply and thus cause paralysis like that in other kinds of stroke.

Bleeding from an aneurysm or angioma may occur spontaneously because of too much thinning of the aneurysm blister or of a blood vessel of an angioma, or because some physical or emotional stress has raised the blood pressure enough to cause the leakage. Occasionally this occurs during pregnancy. Prompt surgical treatment, just as if the patient were not pregnant, usually saves the life of both the mother and child.

Aneurysms: Diagnosis and Treatment

Diagnosis depends ultimately on an arteriogram, which alone can indicate what the trouble is, where it is, and whether or not it can safely be treated by an operation. There are, however, clues that can often establish the true diagnosis before arteriography is performed. Even though an aneurysm seldom gives any advance warning of its presence before it ruptures, the symptoms after it bleeds frequently tell the story. For example, an aneurysm at the base of the skull near the eye nerves (a very common location for aneurysms that bleed) usually leads to enlargement of the pupil of the eye on that side, and drooping of the eyelid. Bleeding from an aneurysm farther forward at the base of the brain, another common site, is more apt to induce mental and emotional changes characterized by drowsiness, poor memory, and confabulation. A bleeding aneurysm tucked into the central fold of the brain, near the nerve cells for sensation and muscle control, can cause numbness and weakness of the opposite arm or leg. Since these symptoms are also typical of other kinds of stroke, it is essential to perform an arteriogram to be certain of the diagnosis.

An example is the case of Mrs. C., a fifty-two-year-old social worker. While quietly eating her supper, she was smitten with a sudden excruciating headache. A few seconds later she lapsed into unconsciousness. By the time the ambulance arrived to take her to the hospital, however, she had revived sufficiently to mumble a few words, complain of headache, and move her arms and legs. At the hospital the doctor, on bending her neck forward, found it to be very stiff, her left pupil was larger than the right, and the left eyelid drooped down over the eyeball. Suspecting a ruptured aneurysm at the base of the brain on the left, he promptly performed a spinal tap, which revealed blood in the CSF. Shortly thereafter arteriography clearly showed an aneurysm where it had been suspected. Mrs. C. was then transferred by ambulance from the local hospital to a large medical center well equipped to treat brain aneurysms.

At the medical center a decision had to be made as to how best to proceed, there being several options.

One is simply to keep the patient in bed for six weeks at complete rest, with enough sedation to keep him a bit drowsy the entire time, so that he never becomes excited or upset sufficiently to raise the blood pressure and thus blow out the aneurysm a second time. If no further bleeding does occur during the six-week period, it can be presumed that healing around the aneurysm has sealed it so well that it may never bleed again, and statistics show that this is often what actually happens. Unfortunately, statistics also show that in spite of this regime, called conservative treatment, there is a 10- to 20-percent chance that the aneurysm will bleed again, usually fatally, about a week or two after the first hemorrhage. Unless such an aneurysm is treated surgically, it is always a threat to life, because it can leak or burst at any time, even years later.

For this reason I believe that surgery is preferable to the program of rest, unless the patient is too old, too weak, or too ill to undergo any type of operation.

There are two methods of surgical treatment. One involves an operation in the neck in order to shut down circulation in the carotid artery that pumps blood directly into the aneurysm. This can be done by tying a thread around the artery (ligation) or by clamping it shut with a small metal device designed for this purpose. The basic principle of this procedure, which is effective for treating some brain aneurysms, is to reduce the direct thrust of blood pumped by the carotid artery into the aneurysm and thus lessen the chance of its rupturing again. The obvious risk of this method is that if the circle of Willis proves inadequate, it may so badly reduce the blood supply that the person may become permanently paralyzed, as if by a stroke. Another risk is that occasionally the aneurysm may burst in spite of this procedure, because the arteries of a fully adequate circle of Willis keep on pumping blood into it.

This operation can be done with safety only if arteriography has shown that the circle of Willis conducts blood in sufficient quantity from the other three main arteries to the brain. If arteriography has shown that the person has been born with a defective circle of Willis that does not carry blood to the side of the brain with the aneurysm, it would then be unsafe to shut off the carotid artery on which that entire side of the brain depends. The only surgical recourse then is an operation directly on the aneurysm itself, inside the skull, which in my opinion is always the procedure of choice provided the condition of the patient is generally satisfactory.

The advantage of an operation on the aneurysm is

that it removes practically all risk of rebleeding without any serious risk of interfering with the circulation to the brain. The operation involves an exposure of the brain similar to that used for brain tumor. The aneurysm is then brought into view by delicate dissection, with the aid of magnification by a binocular microscope or, if this is not available, by magnifying eyeglasses called loupes. During this part of the procedure the blood pressure is deliberately lowered by a special drug given by the anesthesiologist. Lowering the pressure to a safe level in this way for a few minutes causes no harm and greatly reduces the risk of having the aneurysm burst while it is being separated from any surrounding blood and brain tissue that may be stuck to it.

Once exposed, the aneurysm may be treated in either of two ways: coating or occlusion. One method of coating is to apply to the entire surface of the blister a very special liquid, similar to a glue, that hardens as it sticks to the outer wall of the aneurysm. This strong reinforcement of the weak wall prevents any further bleeding. Another equally satisfactory method of coating is to surround every part of the aneurysm with two or three layers of fine muslin. This protects against further leakage and promotes the formation of dense scar tissue all around the blister for additional reinforcement.

The second, and I believe the best, method of treatment is occlusion of the aneurysm by shutting it off completely and for all time by means of little metal clips designed for this purpose, or by a tough thread (ligature) tied around it, where it bulges out of its parent artery. Sometimes a clip or ligature occlusion cannot be done because the aneurysm is simply a large bulge from the artery with no definite stem or neck that can be tied and clipped. This variety therefore requires coating.

The aneurysm harbored by Mrs. C., according to the arteriogram, had a neat stem suitable for clipping and lay near the base of the brain in a quite accessible place. It was therefore decided to perform brain rather than neck surgery and to shut off the aneurysm with a clip. The operation was not scheduled at once, however, because Mrs. C. was still quite drowsy after arriving at the medical center, and it is well known if surgery is performed before the patient has recovered mental and other functions fairly well, these faculties may never be regained. Three days later, when she had become quite alert, surgery was performed as planned, with no difficulty. Later that evening, when fully recovered from anesthesia, she noticed the bandages around her head and remarked to my astonishment: "What did I have? An aneurysm?"

"Yes," I replied, "but how did you know?"

"Because I saw an aneurysm operation on television last week—it was the first thing I thought of. And how glad I am, because I saw how well Ben Casey's patient made out."

Treatment of Angiomas

Angiomas are treated somewhat differently, and again there are two principal methods of dealing with them. The best is to remove them completely from the brain so that there is no longer any risk of bleeding, or of their stealing blood from adjacent parts of the brain that need it. Removal is accomplished by exposing the angioma as for a tumor and then painstakingly identifying and shutting off every one of the arteries feeding blood into its numerous veins. Each artery must not only be shut off by a little metal clip or ligature but then cut in two. For this reason, two clips are placed on each vessel to prevent bleeding from either end, and the vessel is then cut between them. Many of the veins draining an angioma, when first seen, are bright red instead of blue like normal veins. The reason is that blood flows so fast and in such abundance through an angioma that the red arterial blood is pumped almost directly into the veins and colors them red also. As soon as the arteries have been clipped and cut, so that red arterial blood can no longer enter the veins, the latter turn blue. And instead of being enlarged and distended by the blood that was forced into them, they become soft and collapsed. Each vein can now be clipped or ligated and cut, and the whole mass of collapsed blood vessels lifted out.

Mr. Q. illustrates this type of case. He is a young school teacher, twenty-three years of age, who for nearly a year had experienced several shaking fits affecting his right hand and arm, in spite of being given medicines to stop them. Finally he suffered a serious brain hemorrhage similar to that of a stroke. Arteriography disclosed an angioma on the left side of his brain situated just above the location of the speech center and just behind the brain area controlling the right hand and arm.

By the time he was brought to the medical center, he was in fine condition and even eager to have the angioma surgically removed, knowing it could bleed again, perhaps fatally. Following its removal, he resumed teaching and has since married.

Not all angiomas, however, can be removed. Some are too large, occupying most of one cerebral hemisphere. Some are situated in an area, such as a speech center of the brain, that cannot be removed without certain crippling. A few of these can be reduced in size, but not cured, by operating on the brain and shutting off with clips or ligatures their principal feeding arteries. A better method that is sometimes effective is to shut off most of the feeding arteries by artificial emboli consisting of small plastic spheres. Inside each little sphere there is a tiny piece of metal that shows up when x-rays are taken. In this way the precise spot where each sphere lodges in the angioma arteries can be determined. The spheres are injected one by one through a special needle inserted into the carotid artery. Fifty to sixty or more spheres may be necessary to block off the angiomatous arteries, which are studied from time to time during the procedure by injecting, through the carotid needle, a small amount of liquid that shows up in serial angiograms.

Some angiomas are so deep in the brain that they cannot be treated by these plastic spheres unless the spheres are introduced directly into the arteries that feed the angiomas. If one tried to inject spheres through the carotid artery in the neck to treat these deep angiomas, some arteries of other parts of the brain would be blocked off and serious injury would result.

A dramatic new technical development provides for the first time a safe method of sealing seriously enlarged abnormal blood vessels in a deep angioma. This is done by guiding a special tube or catheter into the very mouth of one or more abnormal vessels. Because the main arteries at the base of the brain have a course like the letter S, an ordinary catheter will not pass through their curves.

To solve this problem, the tip of the catheter is magnetically guided through the artery, like a salmon surging up a tortuous river channel. The catheter used is a long, slim, flexible tube having a tiny, perforated stainless steel tip on one end. The steel tip is introduced into a carotid artery in the neck and then guided, by two carefully controlled electromagnets outside the head, inside the carotid artery up to the abnormal brain artery to be treated. One magnet, activated by rapid oscillations of its magnetic field, causes the steel tip to vibrate from side to side, much like a fish's tail, and thus swim, without sticking, around the S curves of the artery. The second magnet, by a steady pull, promotes the upward progress of the catheter, which is also gently pushed by the surgeon or radiologist who is performing the procedure. The desired placement of the tip is confirmed by injecting through the tube a small amount of liquid, which shows up on x-ray film, to outline the blood vessels of the brain and the position of the catheter tip. Artificial emboli may then be introduced through the catheter into the abnormal artery to seal it. This procedure has already proved useful in treating patients.

A new clotting agent now under experimental investigation may eventually prove to be an even better way of sealing these abnormal vessels, by injecting it through this magnetically guided catheter. Another application of this ingenious technique, which originated in Israel, may be the healing of aneurysms by clotting the blood within them by a radio-frequency current induced at the steel tip, once it has been properly positioned.

Rehabilitation of Stroke Victims

The fact that a person suffers a stroke does not necessarily mean permanent paralysis. An elderly friend recently lost all power in her right hand and arm. The paralysis occurred suddenly, with no warning and without any other symptoms such as numbness or speech difficulties. Three days later she regained almost full power in the hand and arm. Clearly the trouble was caused by sudden blockage of the tiny brain artery that nourishes just that part of the motor cortex concerned with hand and arm movements. The blockage could have been due to a spontaneous clot or thrombus inside the artery (a thrombosis) or to a tiny blood clot carried to the artery from the heart or from the carotid artery in the neck (an embolus). Her recovery means that one of three things occurred: a clot spontaneously dissolved, perhaps aided by anticoagulation therapy: an embolus moved on and thus reopened the vessel; or neighboring arteries brought in enough blood past the point of blockage to restore nerve cell function.

Persons who do not recover fully from a stroke may

suffer lasting paralysis or impaired speech, but even for them the future is much brighter than it once was. Rehabilitation efforts often prove highly rewarding in improving or even restoring such lost functions to a useful degree. Experts in the field of rehabilitation medicine have now perfected various ingenious exercises and devices to help people walk or use a partly paralyzed hand, while speech therapists can work wonders in teaching many stroke sufferers how to express themselves again. This is another development that, along with improved surgical techniques, has made the problem of strokes far less dismal than it used to be.

8

Hydrocephalus

One of the most distressing experiences in the life of a physician is to see a child who has something wrong with the brain or the nervous system. It is some comfort, however, that children are not often so afflicted and that when they are many of them can be cured by neurosurgery. Most of these afflictions, popularly known as "conditions," are the result of something a baby is born with.

Perhaps the most familiar is hydrocephalus, or water on the brain, a relatively rare condition caused by increased fluid pressure within the head. In babies and young children, the group most often afflicted, the skull bones have not grown solidly together. Therefore this fluid pressure from within can push the soft bones of the skull so far apart that the whole head becomes grotesquely enlarged. As a rule, hydrocephalus does not become apparent until a few weeks or months after birth, but a few babies have enlarged heads before they are born and may therefore have to be delivered by Caesarian section. The fluid pressure from hydrocephalus can eventually damage the brain and may even be fatal unless surgically treated.

Skull Malformation in Children

The mechanics of skull growth explain why the head may become too large as a result of hydrocephalus. As mentioned earlier, the skull of a newborn baby is made up of islands of cartilagelike tissue. Because these are not yet joined, a certain amount of resiliency exists, allowing for easier birth process and less chance of severe head injury to infants. The moldability of an infant's head is illustrated by the fact that certain primitive tribes in various parts of the world have deliberately changed the shape of their babies' heads. This is done by keeping the infant's head strapped to a board for a year or so. The back of the head then becomes flattened, while the top of the head, pushed upward, becomes abnormally high. This kind of alteration of the skull does not hurt the child or affect the normal development of the brain.

As a normal child grows, the soft islands of the skull become larger, thicker, and harder and then solidly locked in place by teethlike growths along adjacent bone islands. This process of solidification is completed around the age of twenty-one. However, two things can go wrong and adversely affect the size of the head during the early stages of skull growth. One is premature craniosynostosis, too early closure of the cranial bones, a condition which leads to a small, and perhaps deformed, head. Premature closure is a rare condition that can cause brain damage unless surgically corrected. If the skull bones close up solidly before the brain has grown to its normal size, the brain will literally become boxed in, so that it cannot grow and develop as it should. The remedy, which is fairly simple, involves surgery to make cuts in the skull bones that du-

plicate the natural separations between them. This allows
the expanding brain to push the bones apart in a normal
manner as it grows.

The other and more common adverse development
is hydrocephalus, which means that there is an abnormally large amount of the natural fluid (CSF) that exists
within and around the brain and spinal cord in all of us.
It may build up pressure because too much of it is pro-
duced, or because channels through which it naturally
flows have become blocked so that it is dammed up inside the head, or because any excessive amount of it is
not properly absorbed and carried off by the circulating
blood. (In adults this fluid pressure does not enlarge
the head, as in infants and young children, because an
adult's skull bones have joined solidly together.)

Anxious parents often ask whether their child's affliction was any fault of theirs. It probably is not, although
a mother's indulgence in dangerous powerful drugs during
the early life of the embryo may possibly lead to develop-
mental defects, of which hydrocephalus could be one.
Drugs can pass from the mother's blood to the embryo
and prevent its normal development. It is also possible
that a mother's serious illness during the first weeks of
pregnancy could cause hydrocephalus. By and large,
though, the kind of hydrocephalus that a baby is born
with is due to some unfortunate unknown prenatal mischance, possibly genetic and therefore known as a congenital or inborn defect.

Considering the highly complicated and exquisitely
delicate growth of an embryo, it is remarkable that there
are so few aberrations in the development of the human
brain. From the very moment that two cells merge to
start embryonic life, an orderly system of programming
begins. Based on genetic codes in the chromosomes, this
programming leads to the formation of all the very different kinds of cells that make up the body, including

the billions of nerve cells of the brain. Each kind of nerve cell for each part of the brain has its own calendar of development. This calendar can be badly upset if anything goes wrong during the critical early stages of fetal growth. If the pregnant woman has measles at a certain time, for instance, the baby may be born with defective eyesight, while a drug like thalidamide may prevent normal growth of the arms and legs. The same principle undoubtedly applies to the fluid system of the brain—if something goes wrong on the calendar day or days when its channels are developing, they may become blocked or malformed in such a way as to cause hydrocephalus. Hydrocephalus, however, may simply occur because of an inherited or chance fault in the genetic code for brain-cell development.

A serious problem related to hydrocephalus is whether or not there is any associated brain damage. In some cases, for example, the same genetic mischance that has caused the hydrocephalus may also have led to faulty development of the brain. In other cases the enlarged head of the baby may have made the birth process difficult and resulted in brain damage during delivery. Finally, the effect of too much fluid pressure may itself have caused brain damage. The type and degree of brain damage, if any, are determined by the overall evaluation of all the doctor's examinations and tests.

Diagnosis of Hydrocephalus

In infants and young children the diagnosis of hydrocephalus is usually made on finding that the head is too large at birth or that it has begun to enlarge beyond the norm at a later date. The first indication of abnormal head size, however, may not be detected until head measurement, which should be taken at birth and at regular intervals thereafter, show a disproportion between the head and other body dimensions, of which chest size is the most important.

Another simple routine test with infants is to inspect and feel the apertures between the skull bones. The largest of these is the anterior (forward) fontanelle (opening—literally, little fountain) at the top of the head. If it looks and feels tight, instead of soft, this is an indication of pressure inside the skull. Hydrocephalus is the most likely cause of this pressure, although a collection of blood from a hemorrhage over the surface of an infant's brain is another possible cause. If blood is present, it can usually be withdrawn by simply passing a needle through a fontanelle, or if this fails, by a small brain operation.

A third classical test for hydrocephalus, named the Macewen sign after the famous Scottish surgeon Sir William Macewen (1848–1924), is to tap the head sharply but gently with a finger tip. A peculiar hollow sound, known as a cracked pot sound, indicates hydrocephalus of an advanced degree.

The behavior of an individual who is developing pressure in the head may be another indication of hydrocephalus, even though in some cases the head is not enlarged. In an infant pressure generally causes a slowing up of normal reactions; in a child or an adult the ability to think and respond in a normal way is impaired. A baby, for example, may fail to crawl or walk at the expected age and, as pressure progresses, may lose his appetite and even vomit his feedings. Finally he may become listless and drowsy. These are major danger signals. In adults, the diagnosis is indicated by symptoms of increased pressure in the head—headaches, nausea, drowsiness, and failing vision being the most common.

If parents have any doubts about the development of a baby or child, a pediatrician or internist can conduct tests to determine whether anything is really wrong or whether the child simply happens to be one who naturally develops more slowly than others. If there is still any doubt, there are a number of tests, such as I.Q. and other special tests, that can indicate whether an infant, child, or adult is below par with respect to behavioral, physical, and intellectual development.

When hydrocephalus is suspected, diagnostic tests are carried out to confirm its presence and cause and to indicate the best method of treatment. These tests, as well as the various ways of treating hydrocephalus, are all related to the cerebrospinal fluid. This fluid, in addition to surrounding and bathing the brain and spinal cord, fills the four natural cavities, or caverns, deep inside the brain called its ventricles. Too much CSF distends the ventricles and results in increased fluid pressure inside the head.

A major key in the diagnosis of hydrocephalus is proof that these ventricles are enlarged. They are no longer "caverns measureless to man," for their dimensions can now be accurately determined. An arteriogram and an echo-encephalogram, like those used for the diagnosis of a brain tumor or stroke, may reveal evidence of ventricular enlargement. The most effective test, however, is an air test. As mentioned earlier, this requires replacement of some of the fluid in the ventricles with enough air or "contrast" material to show up on x-ray films. Air shows up as a black shadow that reveals the silhouette or outline of the ventricles and thus reveals their size as well as the location of any obstruction of CSF flow. Air is usually introduced directly into a ventricle by a small metal or plastic tube passed through a dime-sized opening in the skull. This is called a ventriculogram. An alternative method, used only when there is no evidence of high pressure in the head, is to introduce air through a lumbar spinal needle and let the air bubble up around and inside the brain—a pneumoencephalogram or PEG. An additional test, also useful for documenting ventricular enlargement and the point of CSF blockage, is a radioactive brain scan similar to that used for the detection of brain tumors. In this case, however, the small and perfectly safe amount of radioactive material is introduced directly into the CSF of the spine by a spinal needle or directly into the ventricular system.

Deciding on Treatment

If infants, children, or adults are perfectly normal until they develop hydrocephalus, their behavior, or in the case of adults, their intellectual capacity, can be restored to its usual level by relieving the fluid pressure on the brain, provided the pressure is relieved before it has caused irreversible brain damage. The results of treatment in this group are generally excellent.

The most agonizing problem and the unhappy side of the coin is whether to treat the infant or child with advanced hydrocephalus—one who has a huge head and severe mental retardation. Some experts strongly advise corrective surgery for this category of patients on the grounds that it enables a child to eat and move about normally and thus makes his care at home or in an institution easier and far less expensive than it otherwise would be. Corrective surgery, they find, may even enable a few children with advanced hydrocephalus to manage three or more years of school. Without corrective surgery, these cases would be doomed to complete invalidism and sure death. This is why some parents insist on every effort to treat the condition, bleak though the prospects for improvement are.

Some Methods of Treatment

Most of the CSF is formed, as a continual self-renewing process, by slim strands of tufted tissue along the floor of each of the four ventricles of the brain. (A small amount of CSF seeps out of the brain itself.) The tufted tissue, which looks like delicate pink seaweed, is called the choroid plexus. Normally, the total amount of CSF in and around the brain and spinal cord would just about fill a drinking glass. Occasionally, however, the choroid plexus, like skin that perspires profusely, secretes much more than this amount. The result is one variety of hydrocephalus—a kind that can be cured by surgically destroying the overproductive choroid plexus.

One way of doing so is to make a small opening in the brain, near the back of the head, where this can be safely done. This small opening is extended down through the brain, on each side, until the two lateral ventricles, which run from front to back inside each half of the brain, are opened. This exposes the choroid plexus at the bottom of each ventricle, which can then be destroyed by an instrument that produces heat from an electrical current at its tip (electro-cauterization). Since the two lateral ventricles are by far the largest of the four, they contain the greatest amount of the choroid plexus. Its obliteration can therefore reduce the production of CSF sufficiently, in some cases, to cure this type of hydrocephalus.

Another method of destroying the choroid plexus is to make two small openings at the back of the head and introduce a small metal tube into the interior of first one and then the other lateral ventricle. This is quite easy, for the ventricles in hydrocephalus are unusually large because of their expansion by CSF. Through the tube, an instrument is inserted that is fitted with an eyepiece at its outer end and a miniature magnifying lens and light at its inner end. With this instrument, called a ventriculoscope, the surgeon can see the choroid plexus and then cauterize it. (One of these ventriculoscopes is on permanent display in the medical section of the Smithsonian Institution, Washington, D.C.)

All the CSF that is formed inside the two lateral

ventricles can escape only through a small opening into
the next or third ventricle—a much smaller, slitlike cavity at the base, or undersurface, of the brain. If a tumor
blocks or obstructs this opening, both lateral ventricles
will become distended because CSF keeps on forming
within them and cannot escape. This is one variety of
what is called obstructive hydrocephalus. It can be treated
by opening a dilated lateral ventricle and removing the
tumor.

The only way fluid can escape from the third ventricle, in turn, is through an extremely narrow tubular
channel at its back end; this is called the aqueduct of
Sylvius after the sixteenth-century French anatomist
who first described it. Our lives hang on this threadlike
channel, less than an inch in length with a caliber as small
as the lead in a pencil. Therefore, the least thing, such
as narrowing from a birth defect, inflammation from infection or bleeding, or compression by an adjacent tumor,
can shut it off. A rapid build-up of fluid pressure in the
dammed-back third and lateral ventricles will then take
place. Blockage in a few cases of this sort can be relieved
by removing the offending tumor or by shrinking the
tumor with x-ray therapy. X-ray treatment, for example,
is often effective for shrinking rare tumors of the pineal
gland, which lies directly above the canal. In a few cases,
it is possible to relieve blockage of the canal by operating
at the back of the head and slipping a small, short, flexible
tube up through the canal, into the third ventricle. The
other end of the tube is placed in a CSF channel just
outside the last, or fourth, ventricle at the base of the
brain. CSF can now flow freely to channels around the
brain where it can be absorbed in a normal way. The
tube, of course, is left in place for the rest of the person's
life, in order to maintain continual CSF drainage from the
third and lateral ventricles. Such a tube is well tolerated,
as illustrated by the case of a boy on whom I performed

such an operation nearly twenty years ago. He thereafter was graduated from school and college and is now a successful business man.

Young H., then fourteen years of age, had been referred to my office because of rapidly worsening headaches, failing vision, and nausea—typical symptoms of increased pressure in the head. On examination, the only things I found wrong were a congested appearance of the optic nerves, discovered by looking into his eyes with a special instrument for this purpose, an inability to move his eyes in an upward direction when asked to look at a fly on the ceiling, and a peculiar hollow sound on tapping his skull with the tip of my finger. The congested eye nerves clearly indicated increased pressure in the head, while the peculiar hollow sound is a characteristic sign of expanded ventricles from hydrocephalus. His inability to look upward was an almost certain explanation of the cause of his hydrocephalus—a tumor of the pineal gland. This is a small gland, normally about the size of a lima bean, which is situated directly above the most forward part of the brainstem. A tiny cluster of nerve cells in this part of the brain governs the muscles that move the eyes upward. Tumors of this gland, which are fortunately very rare, enlarge its size so much that pressure is exerted upon these nerve cells which prevents them from functioning. Immediately below these cells, moreover, lies the slim CSF channel, the aqueduct of Sylvius. A pineal tumor can therefore also press down and shut off this little channel. Consequently the dammed-back CSF will build up inside these ventricles and expand them, thus accounting for the hydrocephalus and increased pressure in the head. X-ray and other special tests that have been described confirmed the hydrocephalus and the pineal tumor causing it.

X-ray treatment usually shrinks and cures such tumors, but not until four or five weeks after treatment is begun. Since only a small amount of x-rays can be safely beamed to the tumor at one time, a patient has to be treated by only a small x-ray exposure each day over a period of four to five weeks. This young boy would almost certainly have died from high pressure in the head in this interval, unless the pressure was surgically relieved. The high pressure could also damage the optic nerves and cause him to go blind. It was therefore imperative to operate promptly and relieve the increased intracranial pressure before starting his course of x-ray therapy. I therefore operated at the back of his head, in order to slip a small tube up through the fourth ventricle and blocked aqueduct of Sylvius into the third ventricle. As soon as the tube entered the third ventricle, clear CSF gushed out of the tube, showing that fluid drainage was now accomplished. The outer end of the tube was then anchored by a sling-like stitch just outside the fourth ventricle, at the very back of his head, where it could continue to drain CSF. The muscles and then the skin were finally stitched together again.

On recovering from anesthesia, the lad no longer had any of his former headaches, and a week later x-ray therapy was begun. He was no longer nauseated, the congestion of his eye nerves cleared up, and the peculiar hollow sound on tapping the head disappeared. As previously stated, he recovered fully, with the exception that he has never regained the ability to look upward—obviously because the nerve cells for this purpose had been permanently damaged by the pressure of the tumor.

By-Passing Procedures

In the case just cited, the blockage of the CSF was relieved by a direct method of draining fluid—that is, by passing a tube directly through the blocked channel. There are, however, other ways of relieving the pressure, by what are known as indirect or "by-passing" procedures. In these the blockage is allowed to remain, usually because it is so extensive or so dangerously situated that it would not be safe to attempt a direct passage of a tube through it. Instead, the fluid is detoured or by-passed around the point of blockage. One way of doing this is to place one end of a small flexible catheter in a distended lateral ventricle. The other end of the tube is then slipped through the vein directly into the small upper right chamber (the atrium) of the heart. This is called a ventriculo-atrial (VA) shunt. CSF will now drain directly into the circulating blood. The shunt tube is fitted at each end with a small valve and, for emergency use, a miniature pumping device that remains buried beneath the scalp. The valve permits just the right amount of CSF drainage. The pump, which can be felt through the scalp, is a flexible compressible little bag about the size of a dime. If headache or drowsiness occurs, indicating that pressure is building up in the head because the tubing has become plugged for some reason, the doctor, or even a member of the family, can press on the pump a few times to force fluid through it and reopen the tubing. If pressure is not promptly relieved, the patient should be taken to a hospital at once. In some cases the outer end of the by-pass tube is placed in the chest outside the lungs, in the abdominal cavity, or in one ureter (the tube that drains the kidney), where CSF can also be readily absorbed, instead of in the heart.

Normally, CSF flows through the aqueduct of Sylvius into the fourth ventricle, at the very back of the head. It drains CSF into the fluid-filled spaces surrounding the brain and spinal cord through three slitlike openings. Plugging of these slits, which is sometimes caused by an inflammation, is another cause of obstructive hydrocephalus. This too requires a by-passing procedure like one of those just described.

What happens to the cerebrospinal fluid after it has flowed out of the fourth ventricle and envelopes the brain and spinal cord like a water jacket?

Outside the ventricles the CSF bathes the entire brain and spinal cord by filling the space between the two delicate transparent inner membranes that cover them: the arachnoid membranes. This fluid-filled space, known as the sub-arachnoid space, continues all the way down the spinal canal as a single fluid system. The pressure within the spinal canal, while a person is lying on his side, will therefore be the same as that in the head. This fact is useful for finding out whether a person really has high pressure in the head, which can be determined by pressure measurements during a spinal tap like that used for a myelogram.

The disposal of CSF is a constant natural process that obviously just keeps pace with its rate of formation, thus maintaining a normal pressure range compatible with life. The principal route by which CSF is finally absorbed within the skull is through little tufts of the arachnoid membrane that surround and open into the veins that drain blood from the brain. These tufts are called arachnoid granulations, or villi.

If the villi become plugged by disease, the CSF cannot escape fast enough and therefore fluid pressure builds up inside the head, resulting either in congestion (edema) and consequent swelling of the brain or in an excessive collection of CSF over the brain and within the ventricles that leads to hydrocephalus. A by-passing procedure is then necessary.

Another, but less effective, route by which CSF escapes is through the sleevelike coverings of brain and spinal cord nerves. This is one reason nerve specialists inspect the interior of the eyeballs of their patients. If the CSF pressure inside the head is too high, this can be detected by a swollen, congested appearance of the optic nerves when they are examined by an ophthalmoscope, or "eye-scope." (Infants and young children with hydrocephalus seldom develop congestion of their optic nerves because their soft skull bones allow the head to expand, which tends to relieve CSF pressure that would otherwise affect the optic nerves.)

Spinal Cysts Related to Hydrocephalus

A fairly common congenital affliction that is sometimes associated with hydrocephalus, although it may occur separately, is a bulging from the spine, usually at the lowermost part of the back. Such a cyst or -cele results from defective closing over the spinal bones long before the baby is born. The membranes called the meninges which cover the spinal cord (myelo-) and its nerve roots, become filled with CSF. The cyst is therefore called a meningomyelocele. If the nerves in it, or the spinal cord (as in some cases), are badly stretched by the bulging and therefore damaged, the infant's legs, bladder, and rectum will be weakened or perhaps paralyzed. The remedy is to operate to reduce the size of the bulge and tuck the nerves (or cord) back in place where they belong. Sometimes this improves leg and bladder control, but too often improvement is impossible.

Results of Hydrocephalus Treatment

It seems worth repeating that the results of treating hydrocephalus are usually excellent if the brain is normal and has not been damaged by defective development, a birth injury, the effects of prolonged fluid pressure, or any other disease process. If there is brain damage, however, correction of the associated hydrocephalus will not restore normal brain function. In some cases of this sort, the alleviation of pressure may improve performance, although never to a normal degree. Based on the experience of many clinics in this and other countries, the surgical treatment of hydrocephalus leads to improvement in 70 to 80 percent of all cases—and some of these cases have now been followed up for as long as thirty years.

A serious drawback, however, is the fact that the majority of patients treated by a by-pass, or shunting, procedure are forever dependent on the functioning of the shunt. Only a few become adjusted to their CSF fluid system so that they no longer have hydrocephalus and no longer depend on their shunt. Shunt dependency is serious because the shunt tubing often becomes plugged—sometimes a few weeks after surgery and sometimes a year or more later. When this happens a second operation—called a revision of the shunt—is generally necessary at once. And some cases require as many as seven or eight revisions. Altogether, about 50 percent of all cases at some time or another require a shunt revision. This points up the obvious need for more effective methods of treatment, a problem that many neurosurgeons are working on. It also indicates the importance of careful regular checkups on every patient, even to the extent of repeating air studies and brain scans in some cases, to see if there is any unsuspected excess of pressure on the brain.

9

Pain

Man's sensory experiences have been a subject of interest and speculation from the time of Plato and Aristotle to the present. Yet it is only in the last hundred years or so that sensations, including that of pain, have been sorted out from one another and their nerve pathways, part of the "wiring system" of the body, charted in blueprint form. As a result of these studies, many features of pain, familiar to all of us, have been made clearer and many different ways of relieving persisting pain have been discovered.

Although most people think of pain as bad, it can also be good, for it is often a first line of defense that protects us from any real harm. It causes us, for instance, to jerk our hand off a hot stove before our fingers get badly burned and warns of appendicitis in time for life-saving surgery. Pain, therefore, is essentially a protective sensation, in contrast to sensations of warmth, cold, and body positions, which are essentially informative.

Almost every part of the body is sensitive to pain, with the exception, paradoxically, of the brain itself. The wiring system for pain is basically similar to that for other kinds of sensation and consists of a vast network of delicate nerve fibers. Their raw ends in the covering, or cornea, of the eyes and in the teeth, skin, and other body tissues are sensitive to anything that irritates them. This is why a cinder in your eye or the touch of a dental drill inside a tooth is painful.

The Relay of Pain

As soon as nerve ends are stimulated, their electrical charge and chemical composition is instantly altered. This alteration immediately evokes a train of similar changes that travel, like an electric current, along the nerve fibers to the spinal cord—the cable that links the body's nerves to the brain.

There are two kinds of pain fibers. The larger in diameter, called A fibers, transmit signals at speeds of up to eighty miles an hour and account for the instantaneous reaction that makes you jerk your hand off the hot stove. The smaller or C fibers, however, send their pain messages at only four miles an hour or less and account for the hot aching feeling, or "slow pain," that persists for some time after a burn. (Other nerve fibers, such as some of those which activate muscles, transmit signals at much greater speeds.)

All the pain fibers from a given part of the body join with other neighboring nerve fibers to form a nerve. When pain signals, or, for that matter, any other kind of sensory signals, reach the spinal cord, they are relayed to the brain by a second set of nerve fibers inside the cord. The brain then sorts out the messages and sends back appropriate commands to muscles, glands, or other body structures through descending nerve fibers in the cord, called motor fibers. Motor signals are then relayed by nerve cells in the cord to motor fibers of the nerves. Thus there is a two-way street for nerve messages. Incoming signals convey information; out-going signals tell body structures such as muscles and glands what to do—either to take action or else to relax by refraining from action, a process known as motor inhibition. There can also be sensory inhibition. A familiar example is the alleviation of minor, local pain by rubbing or scratching the skin. The rubbing sends so many sensory messages along nerve pathways that pain signals are partly blocked. The result is like crossed telephone wires over which three parties are trying to talk at the same time. No messages come through clearly.

The spinal cord not only relays messages up to the brain but also has local relays, through nerve cells, for signals that go directly back to an arm or leg that has sent them. These local cord relays account for reflex action, the reason your hand may be automatically jerked from a hot stove before your brain quite realizes what has happened.

The principal receiving stations in the brain for pain, as well as for other sensations, are two egg-shaped clusters of nerve cells, one in each side of the brain, the right and left thalamus. These are structures deep down inside each cerebral hemisphere. The right thalamus receives messages from the left side of the body, and the left from the right side. This is because sensory fibers cross over from one side to the other—those for pain and temperature perception within the spinal cord and those for other kinds of sensation up in the brainstem at the back of the head. Each variety of sensation has its own domain in the thalamus, and it is there that pain is first consciously appreciated. The nerve cells of the thalamus for pain not only have many connections with other parts of the brain but are also intimately connected with adjacent cells concerned with automatic emotional reactions such as laughing and crying. This is one reason why pain can make us cry so readily. It also explains what happens when a small stroke destroys part of the thalamus and upsets both sensory and emotional control. The victim of such a stroke suffers constant severe pain over the entire opposite side of his body and in addition bursts out from time to time into uncontrollable and utterly inappropriate fits of laughter. This rare condition is known as a thalamic syndrome —syndrome being a term for a constellation of symptoms.

Pain, like other sensory messages, is relayed from the thalamus to higher portions of the brain—the cerebral cortex, or surface gray matter—where there are definite areas for the receipt and interpretation of the various sensations. The major area is the sensory cortex of the parietal lobe, immediately behind the motor cortex, on each side of the head. The thalamus is also connected with other parts of the brain, including the innermost portion of each frontal lobe, which has a great deal to do with emotional feelings. This frontal area of the brain, therefore, plays a role in the psychological rather than the purely automatic emotional responses to pain.

Reactions to Pain

Various factors—psychological, physiological, and physical —influence an individual's reactions to pain. Some people, for example, are born with a low sensitivity for pain and seldom let it bother them. There are even a few rare persons who are totally insensitive to pain except in the cornea of the eye. Others, however, are highly sensitive even to the slightest degree of pain. In still other people, the response to pain—an important factor in pain—may be either blunted or sharpened by environmental circumstances or by their immediate emotional state. Children who have been brought up by brutal parents and beaten regularly sometimes become so accustomed to pain that it ceases to bother them much. Similarly, boxers and football players learn to endure bruises and blows that would tie most of us into knots of pain. On the other hand, children who have been fussed and cooed over every time they suffer the slightest bit of pain may grow up to be adults supersensitive to even trivial discomfort. These are illustrations of conditioning to pain.

Mental and emotional states may also affect the pain response. An athlete is apt to be so engrossed in a game that he does not feel pain until the match is over—a phenomenon that I have personally experienced in my football and boxing days. And someone who is badly upset by business or family worries may at such times be far more sensitive to pain than at any other time—another example of a psychological factor in pain.

Physiological factors must also be considered. Anyone who has walked barefoot on a rocky beach knows how painful this can be for the first few days. But then the pain either decreases or stops, even though there has been no callus formation which would protect pain nerve endings from the full thrust of sharp rocks. The decrease in pain could, of course, happen because of mental conditioning. The brain may simply be saying to the pain nerves: "Oh, stop annoying me with all those signals. Nothing's doing you any harm!" But the reduction of pain may really be due to what is known as adaptation—a physiological phenomenon in which nerves that are subjected to steady stimulation respond less and less vigorously by adapting to the repetitive stimuli.

An individual's body chemistry can be another physical factor affecting pain response, for there are differences from one person to another with respect to hormones and other natural chemical substances which influence the sensitivity of nerve transmission. Various combinations of the factors that have been described, or any one of them alone, may explain why fakirs can walk barefoot on live coals or sleep peacefully on a bed of nails.

Various things can go wrong with the nervous system and alter the sense of pain. Nerves may cease to function as the result of vitamin deficiency, inflammation, or long-continued, excessive alcohol intake (which can physically damage them). The result is a kind of nerve disease, or nerve pathology, known as neuropathy, which can lead to numbness, with loss of pain perception, as well as to paralysis.

There are also spinal-cord diseases, of which multiple sclerosis is one, that may temporarily or permanently interrupt pain pathways in the cord. Pressure upon the cord from a tumor, slipped disc, or dislocated vertebra may also cause numbness and loss of pain perception.

In the brain, diseases or tumors that destroy pain pathways may abolish all sense of pain on the opposite side of the body. As mentioned earlier, a certain kind of stroke, such as that which injures part of the thalamus, may lead to a constant, exaggerated feeling of pain over the opposite side of the body.

Relief by Interrupting Pain Pathways

With respect to the treatment of pain, everyone who has stubbed a toe, cut a finger, bruised a muscle, or experienced a stomach cramp knows that the resulting pain seldom lasts long and obviously does not require the attention of a neurosurgeon. But really intense and lasting pain—the kind caused by severe neuralgia or certain varieties of cancer—often does require the services of a neurosurgeon.

The safest and simplest way to try to relieve pain in

the legs, trunk or arms, when medicines have failed or are required in such large amounts that the person cannot stay awake, is to inject ice-cold saline solution into the cerebrospinal fluid. This is done by means of an ordinary spinal tap low in the back like that used for diagnostic purposes or for a myelogram. The cold saline chills the nerve fibers for sensations of pain enough to put them out of commission for a matter of days or sometimes for weeks but does not cause paralysis or any other disturbances. If pain returns, as it usually does in time, the procedure can easily be repeated. Unfortunately this method of treatment does not always work. For this reason, and because it does not provide long-lasting relief, a surgical method of relieving pain generally becomes necessary.

A neurosurgeon can relieve various kinds of severe pain, depending on their nature and their location, either by an injection that deadens, or "blocks," a nerve or by an operation that interrupts or otherwise modifies pain pathways of the spinal cord or brain. He knows how to do this because the nerves and pain pathways have all been accurately charted, like the shorelines of a seaport, as the result of years of study by many investigators.

Let us trace these pathways from one end of the body to the other—all the way from the big toe to the forward-most part of the brain—and see where and how they can be interrupted or modified to relieve various kinds of pain.

When you have a painful blister on a big toe or a splinter in it, pain begins as soon as the blister or splinter irritates the local nerve ends that detect pain. The nerve fibers of these raw nerve endings converge on their way toward the spinal cord—in which they end—along with other, parallel sensory fibers. All of them form a sensory nerve, and, as for most parts of the body, there is one for the big toe. If it were ever necessary to relieve pain in this toe by numbing the toe—the price of pain relief—

this could be accomplished by deadening its sensory nerve by an injection of Novocain and then alcohol. (Novocain or an equivalent agent is used first in order to numb the nerve before injecting alcohol, because alcohol by itself would cause severe pain.) The toe would not be paralyzed because the sensory nerve contains no motor or muscle nerve fibers. A disadvantage of such a nerve block is that the effects of the alcohol may wear off after a few weeks or months, in which case the nerve recovers and the pain returns. It is therefore preferable, in some circumstances, to cut the sensory nerve—a procedure known as neurotomy—in order to ensure lasting relief.

A sensory nerve like that for the big toe soon merges with other small nerves in its vicinity, forming an ever-larger major nerve such as the sciatic. A major nerve cannot be deadened or cut to kill pain without knocking out the motor fibers, which would paralyze the muscles supplied by that nerve.

On arrival just outside the spine, every major nerve divides into subdivisions small enough to pass through their designated bony openings along the side of the spine. An important feature of nerve fibers with respect to pain relief is that once they are inside the spine, all the sensory nerve fibers become separated from the motor fibers. Within the substance of the spinal cord they terminate as separate small nerve branches and are then called sensory and motor roots. This arrangement allows a neurosurgeon to cut the sensory roots from a painful zone of the body without causing any paralysis, for the motor roots are entirely separate and are not even touched. Cutting these nerve roots requires their exposure by spinal surgery (laminectomy) similar to that used for removal of a slipped disc. The actual cutting of the roots is technically known as a rhizotomy (from rhiz-, root, and -otomy, cutting). This type of procedure is reserved for relief of pain confined to a specific small area of the body when other methods, such as a nerve block, have failed or are inappropriate.

A neurosurgeon knows the exact level of the spine at which to operate in order to numb a particular part of the body. For relief of pain in a big toe, he would operate at the lowest, or lumbar, portion of the spine, and for relief of pain along a rib, at the spinal level corresponding to that rib, as in the case of Mrs. E.

Mrs. E., an active and intelligent woman in her middle fifties, came to me because of persistent nagging pain along the course of her left fifth rib. She attributed the trouble to an automobile accident in which her spine had been badly injured at the level of this rib. X-rays confirmed a definite although not severe injury of the two adjacent vertebrae at that level—enough to pinch the nerve between them on her left side. She had already been seen by several other doctors and reported that some had tried to relieve her discomfort by medicines; others by prolonged rest in bed; and still others by local heat, deep heat (diathermy), ultrasound treatment, massage, and a back brace. All these efforts, including an attempt to deaden the painful nerve by an injection, had failed to help her. She was finally told by the last doctor who saw her that her pain was entirely imaginary and "psychosomatic."

I believed that the pain was real and that the best way to relieve it was to cut the roots of this nerve that conveyed sensations of pain. I explained that this required a spinal operation which would lead to numbness in the area where she suffered rib pain but would not paralyze her—and that it seemed the best way to give her relief. In her desperate frame of mind, she welcomed this proposal and soon entered the hospital for surgery. At operation, to be sure of relieving the pain, I cut not only the principal sensory root of the painful rib nerve but also the root immediately above and below it. The procedure completely relieved her pain and left only a very small zone of numbness. She remains a grateful patient to this day.

Once they have entered the substance of the spinal cord, the fibers of each sensory root end up next to nerve cells through which all messages of sensation are relayed to the brain. The fibers almost touch the nerve cells but are not physically connected to them. They are separated from the cells by an infinitesimal gap called a synapse. Nerve signals jump this gap by lightninglike electrical and chemical changes that occur as soon as a nerve message arrives at the gap. (Several medicines that relieve pain serve to slow down or dampen the transmission of sensory signals at these synapses.) Nerve fibers leaving nerve cells are always an extension of the cell body and are therefore physically part of the cell.

From each sensory nerve cell in the cord a nerve fiber originates that stretches all the way up to the brain. Fibers for different kinds of sensation are grouped inside the spinal cord in separate compact bundles, called tracts. Those for pain—and also for temperature perception—cross over to the opposite side of the cord before coursing upward to the brain. This tract lies close to the surface of the cord, where it can be cut or otherwise interrupted in order to relieve pain. (Fibers for other kinds of sensation, like those which indicate the position of joints and muscles, course upward on the same side of the spinal cord at which they arrive.)

A good way of relieving pain afflicting a large part of the body, such as an entire leg, is to interrupt the tract of pain and temperature fibers for that leg. This is better than cutting all the sensory nerve roots of the leg, which would render the leg completely numb. Although pain and temperature perception would of course be lost after this operation, this is not a serious handicap as compared with constant severe pain. Other sensations, including awareness of the position of the leg, would not be lost.

The greatest risk of cutting the spinal pain tract—an operation called a tractotomy or cordotomy—is the possibility of paralysis. The risk exists because the motor tract, which conveys messages from the brain down to the muscles, lies very close to the pain tract and might be injured.

The pain and temperature tract is technically known as the spinothalamic tract, because its fibers run from the spine to the thalamus, the major receiving station for pain. Spinothalamic tractotomy is usually carried out at a spinal level between the shoulder blades or else in the neck. Once the spinal cord is exposed, the pain tract is cut with a tiny knife blade.

Another method is a percutaneous cordotomy, a procedure that does not require surgery and in expert hands can be done in only thirty minutes or so. A special needle is introduced through the skin (percutaneously) at one side of the neck, and then, with x-ray guidance, it is passed through one of the openings at the side of the spine until its tip rests in the spinothalamic tract that is to be interrupted. The tract is then interrupted by passing a small radio-frequency current through the tip of the needle to destroy the pain and temperature fibers. This procedure has proved extremely beneficial for the relief of severe pain, especially in older persons so weakened by age or disease that they might not survive a cordotomy. There is again a risk of paralysis, although it is slight in expert hands.

Effective relief of severe pain in the neck, face, or throat may require an operation inside the head (such as that used in treatment of tic douloureux, or trigeminal neuralgia, mentioned in Chapter 5) to cut a nerve or to interrupt the specific pathway responsible for transmitting the pain.

Pain in the neck, such as that caused by a cancer,

can be alleviated by interrupting the upward continuation of the spinothalamic tract in the brainstem, either by surgery or by what is known as a stereotaxic procedure. For this procedure a small opening is made in the skull through which a specially designed probe is passed, under x-ray surveillance, by means of a precision device called a stereotaxic apparatus. The tip of the probe is guided with exquisite precision into the pain tract that is to be interrupted. The appropriate nerve fibers are then destroyed either by local heat, induced by a radio-frequency current passed through the probe's tip or by ultra-cooling (cryotherapy) if a cold-producing type of probe is used.

Certain other painful conditions may require an interruption of the thalamus by a stereotaxic procedure. Finally, the intense emotional distress and anxiety associated with some kinds of pain, such as that caused by some cancers, can often be dramatically relieved by what is known as a frontal or prefrontal lobotomy. This procedure is also used, but only as a last resort, for some kinds of mental illness. Lobotomy is a term signifying cutting part of the lobe—in this case, a frontal lobe of the brain. These lobes, and especially their innermost, or cingulate, portions, deal with emotional reactions that tend to magnify pain. By cutting some of the nerve fibers in each frontal lobe, the emotional charge can be reduced so that the person is no longer bothered by his pain even though, paradoxically, he admits it is still present. It is generally necessary to perform lobotomies on both frontal lobes, either by a small operation above the forehead or by a stereotaxic probe. Interruption of fibers of the cingulate portion of each frontal lobe seems to be the most effective procedure. This is technically called a cingulotomy. Although there is very little risk from these small, or "conservative," frontal lobotomies, they always carry a danger of blunting emotional reactions so much that the patient could become dull, careless, and even incapable of self care.

An unusual kind of lobotomy, and one that I devised, is a parietal lobotomy, meaning the cutting of nerve fibers in the parietal lobe, near the middle of the brain. Here is a summary of a case so treated.

Mrs. R., an extremely active, intelligent business woman of sixty-six, was referred to me twenty years ago for relief of what is known as phantom limb pain. This is an unusually distressing type of discomfort that afflicts most persons to some degree, and a few people to a very severe degree, after they have lost an arm or leg. They feel that the missing limb is still there and that it seems to be moving and twisting about in uncomfortably distorted positions. Sometimes severe cramplike or burning sensations of pain may seem to arise in the phantom limb.

One theory of why this happens is that the damaged cut ends of the arm or leg nerves send in distorted signals that upset the usual activity of the brain's circuits for sensory perception, which then also become badly distorted. Another theory is that scar tissue in the amputation stump irritates the ends of the cut nerves, so that they keep sending an unaccustomed, and therefore confusing, barrage of sensory signals to the brain. It is possible in some cases to abolish these painful sensations by operating on the nerve ends in the limb scar. If this kind of operation is not feasible or fails to provide relief, spinal surgery or a percutaneous cordotomy may offer relief. If pain still persists, as it sometimes does after both these procedures, brain surgery for pain relief is the last resort.

Mrs. R. had undergone an apparently successful operation for a cancer of the left breast seven years before she came to me. One year before I saw her, her left arm had to be amputated because of poor circulation. Her distressing cramping, burning, and postural pains in the phantom limb began three days after the amputation. Nerve surgery at the shoulder was out of the question because of the poor local circulation. A spinothalamic cordotomy had therefore been performed, at another hospital, but with relief for only six weeks.

I suggested another attempt at cordotomy, with the hope of cutting pain fibers that might have been missed. But she refused because of the risk of paralysis. She also refused a frontal lobotomy and other types of brain surgery then available for pain relief, on the grounds that she might possibly suffer personality changes and intellectual impairment that would interfere with her business. She also feared that she might be partially paralyzed or perhaps become subject to epileptic seizures. At this point it occurred to me that her bizarre sensations of pain and posturing might be alleviated, if not abolished, by widely cutting the nerve fibers for arm sensations in the parietal lobe of the brain. My idea was based on the fact that large tumors or strokes, which destroy this part of the brain, abolish all awareness of the opposite arm and leg. I also knew that small operations on part of this lobe of the brain, close to the motor cortex, sometimes afforded temporary relief of phantom limb symptoms. I explained that the parietal lobe, behind the motor cortex, was a large area of the brain which dealt with the receipt, sorting out, and interpretation of all sensations from the opposite side of the body, and that cutting its connections with the deep pain station in the thalamus would have a good chance of relieving her pain and other abnormal sensations in the missing arm. I added that the left leg would undoubtedly also be deprived of its sensations, but that there would be very little risk of any personality or intellectual changes or of epileptic seizures as a result of the surgery. The risk of seizures was slight because I planned only a small cut through the surface of the brain—to reach the nerve fibers of the white matter under the cortex—

near the back of the head and therefore far removed from the motor cortex, where an operative scar could easily lead to epileptic fits.

Mrs. R. agreed to this operation, which I called a subcortical parietal lobotomy. Following it, she was completely relieved of her pain and required no more morphine or other strong medicines. Her personality was not altered, and aside from a temporary weakness and the expected numbness of the left leg, she was not in the least handicapped by the operation. She resumed her usual business activities for nearly two years before finally succumbing to the cancer. Without this pain-relieving operation she would have been denied this two-year period of grace.

Other Surgical Procedures

From head to toe, all the pain-relieving procedures that have been described depend on a single basic principle: an interruption of pain pathways. There are, however, two other and entirely different surgical methods of alleviating certain kinds of pain. One is the removal of the pituitary gland (also known as the hypophysis) for the relief of pain caused by some kinds of cancer. The other is modification of pain pathways by an electrical current.

Pituitary gland removal (hypophysectomy) stops the production of the hormones that this gland manufactures and releases into the circulating blood. When these hormones are no longer present, some cancers—cancer of the breast being a notable example—may cease to grow and even wither away to some extent, with consequent relief of the pain they cause and a significant prolongation of life. Hypophysectomy may therefore be extremely beneficial in certain selected cases, although by no means for all victims of cancer. The selection of a suitable case

hinges on expert medical knowledge based on wide experience, x-ray findings, and special chemical tests of the
blood (hormone assays). A fine young schoolteacher on
whom I recently performed this operation was dramatically relieved of her pain, which had been caused by the
spread of breast cancer to the bones. She no longer had
to be confined to bed, as she had been prior to the operation, and regained weight and strength so that she was
able to resume her full teaching schedule for two years.

The gland may be removed by brain surgery, like
that used for a tumor of the pituitary, or by an operation
through the nose—preferably with the aid of a microscope for magnification as described under Strokes,
Aneurysms, and Angiomas. A few university clinics, moreover, are now equipped with extremely expensive equip-
ment that can focus x-ray beams so accurately and
effectively that the pituitary gland can be destroyed
without any kind of surgery.

Electrical methods of relieving pain are not always
effective and seldom of long-lasting value. But when they
do work, they relieve pain in a most dramatic fashion, as
in the following case.

Mrs. Z., some ten years ago, was referred to our clinic
for relief of constant severe bone pain resulting from a
rare variety of cancer. By the time we saw her, she required so much morphine to achieve relief that she literally could not stay awake. Adopting the technique of
Professor Robert G. Heath of Tulane University, I introduced two thin wires, insulated except at their tips, deep
into the frontal lobe of her brain, close to the third ventricle where there are known circuits concerned with emotional feelings that can influence sensations of pain. On
stimulation with these electrodes by a very small electrical
current, she immediately exclaimed, "Oh, I feel so good—
so good—and no more pain—none."

The effects of this stimulation lasted about ten days

possibly because the current had favorably altered the electrical rhythm of emotional and pain circuits for this length of time or had somehow led to a beneficial change in body chemistry. During this ten-day interval she required less and less morphine, regained her appetite, and felt quite comfortable. When pain then began to bother her again, a second stimulation once more afforded relief, but for an interval of only seven days. Finally, succeeding stimulations became less and less effective, apparently because scar tissue formed around the tips of the wires so that the electrical current could no longer reach the nerve fibers. (This is a known fault of permanently implanted electrodes.) The procedure, however, showed that it is sometimes possible, as Heath had demonstrated, to relieve pain and create a feeling of well being by stimulating certain nerve circuits deep in the brain.

Pursuing this principle further, Professor William Sweet and Dr. Vernon Mark of Boston, as well as Professor José Delgado of New Haven, Connecticut, and others, have devised various other methods of electrically modifying pain pathways to bring comfort to their patients. One method involves the placement of implanted electrodes deep in the brain, near the back of the head, where the spinothalamic tract ends. The outer ends of the wires from the electrodes are then connected to a little box provided with a battery, controls to regulate the current, and a button which the patient can push whenever he wishes to relieve his pain. A similar technique has also been used with electrodes placed over sensory tracts of the spinal cord and even over nerves that transmit pain. Theoretically, pain is relieved by these methods because the electrical current gives rise to signals in nerves, pain pathways, or pain circuits that block pain signals or perhaps induce soothing sensations that preempt those of pain.

These two techniques, hypophysectomy and electrical

stimulation, are examples of continuing efforts to discover new and better methods of alleviating pain without the risk of possible unfortunate complications such as paralysis or personality changes.

Anesthesia for surgical procedures—including, probably, Chinese acupuncture—depends on knowledge of pain pathways and various methods of modifying them. The time-honored and still the most widely used method is putting the patient to sleep or at least dulling the state of consciousness so that there is no awareness of pain. In past centuries this was accomplished either with generous amounts of wine or other alcoholic beverages or by the administration of powerful drugs like opium. Modern anesthesia began with the discovery that ether or chloroform would quickly and with reasonable safety put a person to sleep. Safer and more effective agents are now used, some of which are breathed in and others injected into a vein. Their principal action is on the brain as a whole.

For some operations, such as those on a leg, the lower part of the spine, or the abdomen, the lower half of the body can be numbed by spinal anesthesia, so that no pain is felt. For this, an agent like Novocain that numbs nerve fibers in and around the spinal cord is simply injected into the bony canal of the spine by a spinal tap or lumbar puncture, so that it mixes with the cerebrospinal fluid bathing the nerve branches and the cord.

For comparatively minor surgery, such as an operation on a finger, toe, or tooth, it may be necessary merely to deaden the nerve supplying the structure by injecting the nerve with Novocain or an equivalent local anesthetic.

Acupuncture, which is currently being extensively used by the Chinese for major as well as minor surgery, has created a great deal of interest in the Western world. As described in an article "Acupuncture Anesthesia" by Dr. E. Grey Dimond, in *The Journal of the American*

Medical Association (December 6, 1971), it has been used in China for 2,000 years. Whether it depends on hypnosis (which has been used successfully for childbirth and some surgical operations throughout the world) or on generating sensory signals that block out, mask, or jam pain signals in nerve pathways of the spinal cord and brain remains to be determined.

Acupuncture is carried out by placing a needle under the skin at one or more strategic points known to be effective for stopping pain in a particular part of the body. Sometimes the mere placement of the needle is sufficient, but usually the needle is manipulated by a steady, rapid, up-and-down and twirling motion approximately 120 times a minute. A modern refinement is not to move the needle or needles but to run through them a small direct electric current of 9 volts and 5 milliamperes at about 100 cycles per minute. From eye-witness accounts by Dr. Dimond and other reliable American physicians, there is little doubt that acupuncture is safe, simple, and usually effective. In China operations on the lungs, brain, or abdomen are painlessly performed. The patient is fully awake, able to chat freely, and some may even drink a glass of milk during the operation. It seems reasonable to believe that the nerve mechanism of acupuncture and its possible hypnotic effect will be explained and that its application may find a place in present Western methods of anesthesia.

10

Neuromuscular Disorders

Disturbances or diseases of the brain, spinal cord, or nerves that seriously disrupt the power and control of muscles are known as neuromuscular disorders. The names of some of them, such as Parkinson's disease, cerebral palsy, and multiple sclerosis, are almost as familiar to laymen as to physicians, while others, such as spasmodic torticollis, chorea, and myasthenia gravis, are less well-known.

There are also minor neuromuscular disorders that are not at all serious. In everyday life, for example, nearly everyone has suffered an occasional cramp in a leg muscle or in the stomach, and some people occasionally experience mild fluttering or twitching of an eyelid caused by the fatigue of prolonged eyestrain, or by stress.

Another neuromuscular phenomenon that normal people occasionally experience is an abrupt, split-second jerk of body muscles that sometimes occurs when a person is very drowsy and just about ready to fall sound asleep. It feels as if a switch had been turned off, and I am always reminded of high-school experiments on frog muscles, which not only contract when electrically stimulated but also, as they relax, respond with a split-second twitch the moment the stimulating current is turned off. Something like this may be happening as a final step in the preparation for sleep because one of the many circuits concerned with muscle control has been abruptly switched off in the brain.

These common disturbances, while not caused by any disease, share with the serious disorders an interruption of normal muscular activity—either because something has gone wrong with muscles themselves, or, as happens more commonly, because something has affected the nerves that control the muscles. In addition to controlling the movement of muscles, nerves play a role in maintaining the metabolism of muscles which preserves their volume or size, as well as a role in regulating muscle tone. Tone refers to the degree of tension in muscles, such as that necessary to maintain the spine in an upright position while one is sitting at a desk or standing. Without tone, our spinal muscles would be as limp as a rag and we would crumple to the floor.

If a muscle is deprived of its nerve supply by disease or injury of its nerves or of the spinal-cord cells in which its nerves originate, the muscle will not only be paralyzed but will lose tone, becoming flabby and finally wasting away—a phenomenon known as atrophy, meaning absence (*a-*) of nutrition (from the Greek *trophe,* food). Atrophy does not literally occur from a lack of nutrition—for the muscles continue to be nourished by their blood supply—but rather from defective metabolism when their nerve supply is badly damaged. Atrophy may also occur simply from lack of use and exercise of a muscle. Anyone who has lain in bed or had his leg in a cast for a long time knows how weak, flabby, and shrunken the unused muscles usually become.

There are still other ways in which muscles may be affected by disturbances of their nerve supply. Some kinds of spinal cord or brain disturbances, for example, make muscles terribly stiff, or rigid, because of too much tone—a condition known as spasticity. Multiple sclerosis, for instance, sometimes knocks out nerve fibers high up in the spinal cord that convey signals for leg movements from the brain to the nerve cells low down in the cord. The brain sends two kinds of signals to these cells. One kind evokes activity in the cells that make the muscles move by contracting. When these activating signals are blocked by disease or injury, the legs can no longer be moved and are paralyzed as far as control by the brain is concerned. They may move by themselves, however, causing uncontrollable spasms. This is because another kind of signal, which normally prevents excessive activity of the cord's cells, is also blocked. Lacking inhibitory control by the brain, these lower cells literally go wild and fire off so many signals to the muscles that the muscles become extremely tensed from too much tone, and also subject to spasms.

Too much tone and spasticity can also be caused by damage to this inhibitory system in the brain, which is what happens in some kinds of Parkinson's disease and other somewhat similar neuromuscular diseases characterized by extreme rigidity of muscles.

Brain circuits concerned with muscle control may go haywire in still other ways, causing muscles to develop distressing, uncontrollable shaking movements called tremors, or writhing movements called dystonia (from *dys,* a disturbance of, and *tonia-,* tone).

Control of your muscles—even the apparently simple neuromuscular act of waving your arm—is a highly complicated affair as far as the nervous system is concerned. Apart from nerve circuits for sensations of the arm's position, such control involves a number of major motor circuits. One circuit consists principally of the nerve cells in the area of the cortex called the motor strip. Its cells are responsible for the initiation of arm and other movements of the opposite side of the body.

Deep down in the brain there are other circuits which are largely concerned with the regulation of muscle tone and the smooth coordination of muscular activity. These are circuits in parts of the deep structures of the brain called the thalamus, basal ganglia and brainstem. In addition, there are circuits in the cerebellum, which are also essential for smoothness of muscle performance.

Finally, signals from all these different circuits in the brain converge on the nerve cells of the spinal cord which tell the muscles what to do. The teamwork between all these complex circuits enables one to wave an arm, or a baseball pitcher to throw a fast ball.

Diagnostic measures used to distinguish one kind of neuromuscular disorder from another depend on the history of the illness, a thorough examination of the patient, and various tests such as an electrical recording from muscles (an electromyogram or EMG), special x-ray and CSF studies, and any special blood tests that may be indicated.

Most neuromuscular diseases are diagnosed and treated by neurologists, but certain patients are referred to a neurosurgeon for treatment. This was especially true of victims of Parkinson's disease a few years ago, before the discovery of a new medicine that is now widely used for treating this condition. Sometimes it is still necessary to call upon a neurosurgeon when patients fail to improve with this medicine.

Parkinson's Disease

Parkinson's disease is a fairly common affliction that usually first affects persons when they are around fifty or sixty years old. Although it is an age-old disease, it was not formally described until 1817 when a British physician, James Parkinson, called it "Shaking Palsy."

The first symptoms vary from case to case and sometimes are quite bizarre, as illustrated by the following example. This was a patient who almost got into a fight because a man at an adjacent restaurant table accused him of winking at his girl. The patient had come to me for just that reason: because of an intermittent, uncontrollable blinking of his eyelids—a symptom called blepharospasm. It is a well-known form of spasmodic muscle contraction of the eyelids sometimes, as in this case, associated with Parkinson's disease and is occasionally a first symptom of this disease. Fortunately this patient responded well to treatment by medicines prescribed by the neurologist to whom I referred him.

The more common symptoms of Parkinson's disease consist of insidiously progressive stiffness of the muscles that eventually may make walking so difficult that the victim can only shuffle along. Stiffness of the facial muscles is also common, and may become so pronounced that a normally vivacious person may be unable to smile or demonstrate his usual facial expressions in response to jokes or ordinary conversation. This "dead-pan" appearance is technically known as masking, or a masked face. In addition to muscle stiffness or rigidity, a rhythmic to-and-fro tremor of one or both arms (or the legs and feet) is not uncommon—which makes it impossible to lift a glass of water to the mouth without spilling it. This tremor, combined with the muscle rigidity that partly paralyzes the person, gives rise to the term shaking palsy.

Until relatively recently, the treatment of Parkinson's disease was not satisfactory, although symptoms in some cases could be partially relieved by a medicine called atropine, or by chemically related or synthetic medicines similar to atropine, which restrict the abnormal nerve signals deep in the brain that cause symptoms. This, however, was a clue suggesting that perhaps more effective chemical substances might be found. Another clue was the discovery that a commonly used synthetic tranquillizer, chlopromazine, if taken in too large amounts by a perfectly normal person, would sometimes induce tremors and rigidity like those of Parkinson's disease. A third clue was provided by research directed at finding out more about the chemistry of nerve cells of the brain concerned with the control of muscles, and particularly the cells which regulate muscle tone and coordination. (The chemistry of the brain's nerve cells is not all the same—cells of some circuits have individual chemical peculiarities and needs that are entirely different from those of other nerve cells.) All this research proved that the nerve cells deep in the brain, which give rise to symptoms of Parkinson's disease, require an ample amount of a substance called dopamine. Without this, they fail to transmit nerve signals properly and cause symptoms. Further investigation showed that this substance was deficient when disease, age, poor circulation, or other factors afflicted the deep motor circuits of the brain. Their nerve cells—or what was left of them if some had been destroyed by the disease—could therefore not function. But when patients were given a substance called L-dopa, which restores dopamine, symptoms of Parkinson's disease cleared up.

Several victims of this disease whom I personally know have been severely handicapped for years, some so badly that they were confined to wheel chairs. Yet today, thanks to treatment by L-dopa, they are able to walk, partially care for themselves, and even go to their offices every day.

Through the work of Dr. George Cotzius of the Brookhaven Laboratories in Long Island, New York, who was a pioneer in the discovery of L-dopa, and additional research by Professor Melvin Yahr and his colleagues at the College of Physicians and Surgeons of Columbia University, additional new agents have recently been developed which promise even greater benefits for patients with this disease.

All these agents, however, must be prescribed, and their use carefully guided, by an expert neurologist. This is because, in some cases, they can lead to distressing and potentially dangerous side effects such as very low blood pressure and bizarre mental or emotional disturbances.

If L-dopa or related substances fail to improve symptoms, brain surgery offers hope for improvement. The following case, operated upon before the discovery of L-dopa, at a time when brain surgery was frequently used for the treatment of Parkinson's disease, illustrates how this type of surgery was performed and what it can achieve.

Mrs. O., aged 58, was referred to our hospital because she was bothered by an uncontrollable to-and-fro tremor of her right hand and arm. The trouble had begun with a shaking movement of just the right thumb about a year previously. This tremor then insidiously spread up the right arm until it shook so badly that she could not feed herself without using the other hand and arm. There were no other symptoms.

She proved to be an extremely bright, intelligent woman, with nothing apparently wrong except the tremor and a lack of normal facial expression, which gave her a dead-pan appearance. Unlike many patients with this disease, she suffered no muscle rigidity. An ample trial of appropriate medicines available at that time had not significantly lessened her tremor.

She and her husband were both well aware that she had Parkinson's disease and were of course anxious to know what might have caused the trouble and how she might be helped.

We explained, first, that we did not know the cause but that there were several possibilities. One was poor circulation from premature hardening of arteries in parts of the brain concerned with muscle tone and coordination. Another was either a wasting away—degeneration— of these parts of the brain, or else some local disorder of nerve cell chemistry that put them out of action. Still another possibility was a virus infection of the brain, such as that which causes encephalitis, or "sleeping sickness," and which can lead, twenty years or so after recovery from the attack of encephalitis, to symptoms of Parkinson's disease. This is because some viruses—called slow viruses—may not cause permanent tissue damage until many years after they have infected a tissue of the body.

We then pointed out that brain surgery offered a real hope—but no guarantee—of alleviating her symptoms and of course added that, like any surgery, it always carried a risk of complications, the major risk in this instance being the possibility of paralysis. Since her condition was rapidly worsening and medical treatment had failed, we felt that surgery was her only hope. Before agreeing, Mr. and Mrs. O. quite naturally requested a full explanation of precisely what the operation involved.

We therefore explained that it involves putting a small probe in the brain by what is known as a stereotaxic procedure, described in the chapter on Pain. Technically, this stereotaxic procedure is called a thalamotomy because a portion of the thalamus, one of the deep substations that deal with muscle control, is cut, not with a knife but by a small radio-frequency current at the tip of the probe. When the appropriate segment of the thalamus—and it is only about a quarter of an inch in diameter —is destroyed, tremor vanishes. We also pointed out that a preliminary test called a ventriculogram is required to outline the ventricles of the brain, for they serve as essential navigational landmarks for accurate placement of the special probe used for this operation. They are clearly outlined by x-rays after a small amount of air is introduced by a spinal tap, like that for a myelogram in a person with a slipped disc. The air passes up inside the spinal canal to enter the ventricles. Measurements of the interior of the brain can then be determined with millimeter precision. In some clinics the ventricles are outlined by putting a radio-opaque liquid directly into them, a test known as a contrast ventriculogram.

The actual surgery is relatively minor compared with most brain operations and is performed under local anesthesia with the patient well calmed by tranquilizing medicines. The patient must remain sufficiently awake so that the tremor or rigidity can be tested as proof of correct placement of the tip of the probe. The probe is introduced through a nickel-sized opening made in the skull. The probe, securely held by a well-designed mechanical apparatus attached to the head, is then slowly lowered and carefully guided into the brain.

Thanks to the Novocain in the scalp and the fact that the brain itself is not in the least sensitive to pain when touched or probed, these operations are not at all painful.

When the probe is properly positioned, the desired part of the brain—in this instance part of the thalamus—is completely destroyed, either by a small radio-frequency current or by intense local cooling called cryotherapy, a technique perfected for use in the brain and still used by Dr. Irving Cooper of St. Barnabas Hospital, New York City. Parkinsonian symptoms, although caused by disease of parts of thalamic or other related deep circuits, can be relieved by completely interrupting one or more of these circuits by surgery, which reduces or abolishes the abnormal signals that have been causing tremor or rigidity.

We explained all of this to Mr. and Mrs. O. in relatively simple terms, although of course pointing out the risks. She eagerly welcomed this chance for relief, and accordingly the operation was performed.

All went well, and even before the probe was withdrawn her tremor had vanished—and it did not return in the ensuing period of ten years during which we kept track of her.

Unfortunately, it is not possible to attain such a good result in every case, but sometimes, in our experience and that of others, a second operation will stop a tremor that returns. And in some cases it has been necessary to perform stereotaxic surgery on both sides of the brain to relieve tremor or rigidity on both sides of the body. Today these operations are infrequent because modern medical treatment is so much improved.

Related Disturbances of Muscle Activity

In addition to Parkinson's disease, there are other defects (or lesions) of the basal ganglia which are the cause of uncontrollable movements of muscles, called dyskinesias, meaning disturbances of muscle motions, or muscle kinetics. One form of dyskinesia is athetosis, characterized by almost constant distressing writhing motions of the arms or legs, and usually also of the face. The latter take the form of unpleasant mouthing and grimacing movements. Another kind of dyskinesia is chorea (St. Vitus' dance), which is accompanied by constant, aimless, brisk, but rather graceful contortions of the limbs. In some cases it is caused by an inherited defect of the basal ganglia but in others is caused by rheumatic fever that affects the basal ganglia. In children it usually appears between five and fifteen years of age.

An example of an allied disorder, called dystonia, (disturbed muscle tone) is cited to indicate how its symptoms, like those of Parkinson's disease, can sometimes be dramatically improved by stereotaxic surgery.

Mr. M. was twenty years old when first seen by Dr.

Edgar M. Housepian and me. His trouble may well have been due to some brain damage at birth, for his mother told us the delivery had been difficult.

The first sign of trouble was apparently a gradual loss of control of his right hand when he was five years old. By the time he was fifteen he also developed a peculiar shaking tremor of the opposite or left shoulder, which five years later began in addition to affect his left leg to such an extent that it often caused him to fall. And by the time we saw him his left neck muscles were also so badly affected that they kept jerking, twisting, and rotating his head—a most distressing condition. Since medicines had brought no appreciable relief, he had been referred to us for brain surgery as a last resort.

Stereotaxic thalamotomy, similar to that for Mrs. O., was accordingly performed on the right side of his brain. To everyone's joy, it stopped the dystonic muscle movements of his neck, left arm, and left leg, and they never returned during the nine years of follow-up.

Certain other neuromuscular conditions are characterized by bizarre muscle contractions that are psychologically distressing but not physically serious or incapacitating. A fairly common one is a tic or spasm of the neck muscles. It is called spasmodic torticollis because of periodic twisting or torsion movements of the neck (from Latin *collis*, neck—the word that gives rise to collar).

In this condition, which usually persists through life but seldom gets any worse, the head is pulled abruptly down and to one side until the chin almost bangs the shoulder. Some psychiatrists in the past have considered the condition to be of psychological origin, which started because, for some reason, the person wanted to "look away from life and not face it." The prevailing opinion today is that this type of muscle tic, like those associated with uncontrollable grimacing motions of the face, stems from a small lesion in the basal ganglia or thalamus.

Treatment by tranquilizing medicines seldom helps. One method of treatment—although it seldom stops these tics completely—is surgery to cut some or all of the nerves which supply the affected muscles. Since this operation obviously weakens the affected neck or face muscles, most people prefer to go about their business with their tic.

Cerebral Palsy

Another kind of neuromuscular disorder of brain origin is cerebral palsy. This is a tragic affliction that may be caused by some fault in brain growth before an infant is born or by brain damage at the time of birth. In either case one half (one cerebral hemisphere) of the brain is so poorly developed or else so badly damaged that the muscles of the opposite side of the body become either very weak or almost totally paralyzed. They are also so stiff from hypertonia—because many motor circuits are impaired—that they are spastic. This type of brain damage, in addition, is generally accomplished by some degree of mental retardation, difficulty in speaking, and epileptic seizures.

If medicines and rehabilitation efforts fail to improve symptoms, brain surgery sometimes proves beneficial. It involves removing most or all of the hopelessly damaged half of the brain—which can never have any useful function. This removal (called hemispherectomy), in properly selected cases, sometimes reduces the degree of spasticity so that a child can walk and get around better than before the operation. Other advantages of the operation, if it is successful, include reduction or cessation of seizures and improvement in behavior and intellectual capacity. The improvement occurs because hemispherectomy removes "bad" brain tissue, the source of distorted nerve signals that cause seizures and also disturb the opposite, healthy cerebral hemisphere. When the healthy remaining half of the brain is no longer electrically disturbed, it can function up to its full capacity. This is why intellectual performance may improve. But, sad to say, one can never expect the child to grow up with a completely normal intellectual capacity or ever to regain full use of his already partly paralyzed muscles.

Spinal-Cord Disorders

Among neuromuscular disorders of spinal cord origin, poliomyelitis not many years ago was one of the most common. Today, fortunately, it is a rare disease, thanks to the widespread administration of oral vaccines that usually prevent the infection.

Poliomyelitis (from the Greek *polios-*, gray matter, and *myelitis,* infection of the cord) is caused by a virus that rapidly alters and may even destroy the nerve cells of the spinal cord that move the muscles—the anterior horn cells (in the forward or anterior part of the gray matter of the cord). When these cells are put out of commission or actually destroyed, marked muscle wasting and paralysis occur. Reflexes disappear and the muscles become limp from lack of tone because nerve messages are no longer sent out to them, the nerve cells that normally supply them having been destroyed.

A common, but still unconquered, spinal-cord ailment that leads to neuromuscular symptoms is multiple sclerosis (MS). It may occur at almost any age from childhood to late middle age and may also affect the brain and the optic nerves. It is characterized by multiple spotty areas of hardening (sclerosis) in the spinal cord or brain, which temporarily or permanently injure nerve cells and nerve pathways. The result is temporary or permanent muscle weakness, wasting, or paralysis. In MS there are usually also disturbances of body sensations and perhaps of vision. In many cases symptoms disappear spontaneously after a few weeks, but often they reappear, months or even years later, perhaps in different parts of the cord or brain. In some cases, however, the disease seems to burn itself out, so that new symptoms never again develop.

While the cause of MS has not yet been established, recent studies suggest that it may result from a slow virus infection of the spinal cord or the brain. The theory hinges in part on the geographic distribution of cases of MS, since it is especially prevalent in countries with cold damp climates where virus diseases are prevalent, and in part on experiments with sheep and other animals susceptible to virus infections that produce similar symptoms. There is at present no really effective treatment, with the exception that some cases respond to certain steroids.

Patients with MS (or with ALS, which is next described), should not be under the care of a neurosurgeon, for there is no known surgical remedy for these diseases. Such patients should be cared for by a neurologist, who will be knowledgeable about the newest methods of treatment and research in these afflictions.

Another somewhat similar disease is amyotrophic lateral sclerosis (ALS). The term amyotrophic is made up of the elements *a-*, meaning absent or poor, *myo-*, muscle, and *trophic-*, growth, and really means that there is wasting of muscles. The condition is sometimes referred to as Lou Gehrig's disease, after the famous baseball player of the 1940s, who finally died of it.

The muscle wasting occurs because the disease destroys the nerve cells in the cord from which the muscles' nerves originate. If these cells, which are the anterior horn cells, die as the result of disease, their fibers also die and wither all the way down a nerve to the muscle they supply. Consequently that part of the muscle also dies. It not only becomes paralyzed and loses tone, but actually wastes or withers away.

The terms lateral (side) and sclerosis refer to the fact that in ALS the nerve pathways of one or both sides of the spinal cord, which convey signals from the brain to the anterior horn cells, are destroyed by sclerosis. This is another factor that can lead to paralysis—from interruption of voluntary control over muscles. It can also lead to overactive reflexes because the brain's inhibitory or checking influence on intact nerve cells of the cord is removed.

This disease usually affects people in late middle age and, unlike MS, does not affect the brain or vision or lead to any disturbances in sensation. It tends to be very slowly progressive over a period of many years. The first signs usually are wasting of the hand muscles that move the fingers and a gradually increasing difficulty in walking from weakness and perhaps stiffness (from hypertonia) of the legs. Another typical symptom of ALS is occasional twitching or rippling of affected muscles, called fasiculation because the twitches involve various bundles, or fasicles, of a muscle. They occur because in ALS the anterior horn cells are not destroyed rapidly; consequently, these cells are at first only gradually affected by the disease, in a way that irritates them and makes them fire off random signals. These random signals make related segments of the muscles twitch or ripple from time to time, in an irregular way.

The specialist called upon for the diagnosis and treatment of these spinal diseases must make certain that the symptoms are not caused by some other, curable condition such as a benign spinal tumor, enlarged spinal blood vessels, a slipped disc, some misshapen or thickened spur of bone that can be removed, or the late effects of syphilis

—which sometimes affect the spinal cord as well as the brain.

Faulty Signals from Nerve Cells

Disorders of the nerves themselves may also upset muscle control and power, for when the nerves fail to conduct signals, the muscles obviously will respond either weakly or not at all and will also become flabby and atrophied from disuse and loss of tone.

One condition that occasionally afflicts nerves is neuropathy, meaning a diseased state of nerves. In this condition the nerve's fibers degenerate, in some cases permanently, but in other cases with recovery under proper treatment. The neuropathy may be a result of vitamin B deficiency, the long-continued indulgence in too much alcohol, or a remedial metabolic disorder. Recovery can be achieved by, respectively, treatment with vitamin B, foregoing alcohol, or correcting the error in metabolism. Neuropathy of unknown cause, or the kind that follows exposure to toxic chemicals or certain heavy metals, is usually less apt to be curable.

Neuritis, meaning nerve inflammation, may occur because of a virus or some other infection, or for some unknown reason. It too may lead to weakness or paralysis. (When many nerves are involved, the term polyneuritis is used.) In some cases this condition clears up by itself, but in others it does not, despite treatment by vitamin B, rest, and, if indicated, by antibiotics to combat an infection, or by steroids to allay congestion in the affected nerves.

An entirely different kind of disease is a serious, but fortunately treatable, condition called myasthenia gravis (from *myo-*, muscle, *asthenia-*, weakness, and *gravis-*, grave or serious). It was first described in 1672 by Thomas Willis, discoverer of the circle of Willis mentioned in Chapter 7. This disease is characterized by extremely rapid fatigability of muscles. The eyelids are often affected first, and because of their fatigue, the upper lids droop until the eyes are almost shut. If muscles that move the eyes are affected, blurring of vision will occur because of double vision. And, with rapid and successive movements of the hands, as in repeatedly making a fist, the muscles become so weak that within a minute or so it is scarcely possible to close the fingers. When severe, this disease can weaken the breathing muscles so seriously that respiration by an automatic respirator may be necessary day and night. Neurological specialists tell me, however, that only about 15 percent of all patients afflicted with myasthenia gravis ever require prolonged artificial respiration, and that after medical treatment for three to five years many other patients spontaneously recover from the disease and no longer require any special medicines. Finally, most of those who continue to need the medicines that relieve symptoms are able to lead a normal life for many years with the aid of these medicines.

Mrs. F., an attractive housewife of twenty-nine, was recently referred to my office because of drooping of the left eyelid and double vision that had suggested to her doctor the possibility of a brain tumor or an aneurysm back of the left eye, where pressure on eye nerves can cause these symptoms.

Her trouble had begun four months previously, starting with drooping of the left upper eyelid that at first occurred only late every day and never in the morning. This time factor of her symptoms immediately suggested that muscle fatigue like that characteristic of myasthenia gravis, rather than pressure on nerves, was the cause of the trouble, since pressure on eye nerves from a tumor or aneurysm usually affects these nerves rather steadily and not simply at times of the day when the individual is tired.

Gradually this late-afternoon drooping became worse, and finally, three weeks before I saw her, her eyesight became blurred because of "double vision." At this juncture she had gone to a small eye clinic where she was told she simply had "eye fatigue." She had no other symptoms save for a slowly progressive tendency to tire easily toward later afternoon.

My examination showed nothing wrong with Mrs. F. except for pronounced drooping of the left eyelid, inability to move the left eye as far up and out as the right eye (which accounted for her double vision), and a tendency for all muscles to tire and feel weak very rapidly when vigorously exercised during my testing. These findings, plus her story, were so typical of myasthenia gravis that I referred her at once to one of our expert neurologists who specializes in the diagnosis and treatment of this disease.

He arranged x-rays and other special tests to be absolutely certain she had no tumor or aneurysm and then gave her a small dose of a medicine called Tensilon, which is known to improve muscle function in myasthenia. With almost magical rapidity this medicine resulted in much less drooping of her eyelid and lessening of the double vision. The diagnosis having been established, he then prescribed regular daily doses of another medicine known to be an effective treatment for the weak muscles of myasthenia. Since then she has been practically free of the drooping eyelid, double vision, and the former general fatigue of other muscles.

Myasthenia gravis is a disease caused by faulty transmission of nerve impulses at the synapses where motor nerve fibers end on muscle cells and for this very reason it can often be cured. There are chemical agents that can restore effective transmission at the affected nerve endings, neostigmine being one. In addition, removal of the thymus, a gland tucked under the upper part of the breastbone, also helps to alleviate symptoms in some cases. Removal of this gland probably improves something that is wrong with an immune system that has disturbed nerve-muscle transmission.

Although some neuromuscular disorders can be remedied and a few cured spontaneously, a considerable number defy treatment. Since effective treatment depends on precise knowledge of the cause of the disease, a great deal more research is obviously needed. More research is also needed on ways of preventing the inborn defects of the nervous system that cause some of these diseases. Progress is being made, however, for this kind of work is going on in many laboratories throughout the world. Just recently, for example, new medicines have been developed which dramatically relieve severe muscle spasms, particularly those associated with some of the neuromuscular disorders of children, for which in past years there has been no effective treatment. And there is a growing hope that a cure will eventually be found for multiple sclerosis and some of the other diseases that have been described.

Conclusion

This account of modern brain and nerve surgery illustrates major developments during the span of my medical career which have led to the saving of many more lives and the relief of many more distressing ailments of the nervous system than was possible or even dreamed of forty years ago. At that time, for example, before the advent of antibiotics, most victims of paraplegia from a severe spinal injury died within a year. Today, thanks to antiobiotic therapy and sophisticated methods of treatment by neurosurgeons and other specialists, the long-term survival of such patients is close to 85 percent instead of the 3 percent it used to be.

Victims of certain kinds of stroke likewise can now be saved and in many instances restored to a normal life, thanks to improved neurosurgical techniques. An outstanding example is the relief of stroke symptoms by opening up arteries in the neck that have become so thickened by arteriosclerosis that they no longer carry enough blood to the brain. Forty years ago this kind of surgery was practically unheard of. Today it is common practice, as exemplified by a medical colleague, now back at full work, who recently had both of the carotid arteries in his neck opened by surgery.

Brain hemorrhage from a leaking aneurysm—a condition usually written off as a hopeless stroke thirty years ago—can now be successfully treated by a neurosurgical operation. Even fifteen years ago such operations proved successful in only about 50 percent of such cases, whereas today, thanks to continued research and technical developments, the success rate for this kind of surgery is close to 95 percent if the hemorrhage has not been too severe and the person is in reasonably good condition.

Thirty to forty years ago very few neurosurgeons ever dared to remove completely certain brain tumors, like the noncancerous variety which press on the hearing nerve. Consequently the results of surgery were often poor, and further operations were frequently necessary because the residual tumor grew back. Now, owing to improved methods of both anesthesia and surgery, plus the aid of magnification by special eyeglasses or a binocular microscope, these and other difficult tumors can be totally removed with very little risk of complications.

Another fairly recent development is stereotaxic surgery that interrupts nerve circuits deep in the brain by means of an accurately guided special probe. This is one way of relieving some kinds of shaking tremors or severe pain, when they do not respond to treatment by special medicines. Some kinds of pain can even be relieved by recently devised apparatus which delivers a mild electrical current by wires in nerves or in certain parts of the spinal cord or brain. It has also been found that pain from some kinds of cancer can be dramatically relieved—and life prolonged—by surgical removal of the pituitary gland at the base of the brain. Only in the past fifteen years or so, moreover, have ingenious miniature valves been perfected that can be permanently placed in the head to relieve the dangerous pressure caused by hydrocephalus.

Other developments that I have witnessed are diagnostic tests such as the electroencephalogram, visualization of the blood vessels of the brain and spinal cord by arteriography, and the painless detection of brain tumors by radioactive scanning techniques. These three commonly used tests alone—and there are still others—have made it possible to detect trouble before it is too late and to pinpoint its exact location in the brain or spinal cord.

This brief outline of some of the diagnostic and neurosurgical advances in the past three or four decades indicates, I firmly believe, that research during the next thirty years will be marked by equally splendid improvements which will save more and more lives and may even restore power to crippled limbs and sight to the blind.

Glossary

For Further Reading

Index

Glossary

ADENOMA

tumor of a gland.

ADRENAL GLAND

gland above each kidney that makes adrenaline and other HORMONES.

AIR STUDY

x-ray test in which some of the CERE-BROSPINAL FLUID is replaced by air.

AMNESIA

loss of memory.

AMYTROPHIC LAT-
ERAL SCLEROSIS
(ALS)

a disease of the spinal cord of unknown cause.

ANEURYSM

blisterlike out-pouching of the wall of an artery that may leak blood or burst.

ANGIOMA

cluster of abnormal blood vessels, usually oversized and including arteries and veins that may leak blood or burst.

AQUEDUCT OF SYLVIUS	tiny channel deep in the brain for the escape of CEREBROSPINAL FLUID.
ARACHNOID	thin transparent membranous covering of the brain and spinal cord with spider-web-like extensions.
ARTERIOGRAM	x-ray test which outlines blood vessels for diagnostic purposes.
ARTERIOVENOUS MALFORMATION	condition in which arteries and veins are malformed prior to birth; another term for ANGIOMA.
ASTHENIA	weakness, as in myasthenia, weakness of muscles.
ATHETOSIS	one variety of distressing, uncontrollable muscle movements.
ATONIA	absence of MUSCULAR TONE.
ATROPHY	a wasting away, as of muscles.
AUTONOMIC NERVOUS SYSTEM (ANS)	the predominately automatic system of nerves which helps regulate functions such as heart rate, blood pressure, and digestion.
AURA	sensory experience; in epileptics, sometimes a warning of an impending attack.
AXON	see NERVE FIBER.
BASAL GANGLIA (B.G.)	clusters (GANGLIA) of nerve cells constituting part of the gray deep matter in the brain near its base.
BRAINSTEM	the stemlike extension of the brain which connects it with the spinal cord.

CATHETER	flexible plastic or rubber tube.
CAUDA EQUINA	the crowded collection of nerve connections (NERVE ROOTS) inside the lowermost portion of the spine.
CENTRAL NERVOUS SYSTEM (CNS)	the brain and spinal cord.
CEREBELLUM	the "little brain," smaller and different in shape, appearance, and function from the rest of the brain; it lies under the cerebral hemispheres at the back of the head.
CEREBRAL	pertaining to the brain or the CEREBRUM.
CEREBRAL CORTEX	mantle of nerve cells over the entire surface of the brain that comprises its external GRAY MATTER.
CEREBRAL PALSY	form of PARALYSIS caused by disease or defective development of the brain of young children.
CEREBRAL VASCULAR ACCIDENT (CVA)	stroke caused by blood vessel (vascular) disease or hemorrhage.
CEREBROSPINAL FLUID (CSF)	natural clear watery fluid that bathes the brain and spinal cord and fills the internal cavities of the brain called VENTRICLES.
CEREBRUM	the major portion of the brain, consisting of the two large hemispheres.
CERVICAL	pertaining to the neck.
CHEMOTHERAPY	treatment with chemicals.

CHOREA — a particular variety of involuntary writhing and twisting movements of muscles.

CHOROID PLEXUS — pink tufted tissue inside the VENTRICLES of the brain, which forms most of the CEREBROSPINAL FLUID.

CINGULOTOMY — form of LOBOTOMY in which nerve connections of the cingulate gyrus or CONVOLUTION of one or both frontal lobes of the brain are cut or otherwise interrupted.

CIRCLE OF WILLIS — circular arrangement of interconnecting major brain arteries at the base of the brain.

COCCYX — last bone, or "tail" bone, of the spine.

COMA — state of profound unconsciousness.

CONCUSSION — temporary loss of nerve function without any perceptible permanent damage or loss of function, caused by a sudden blow; may affect the brain, spinal cord, or a nerve.

"CONDITION" — term popularly used to indicate symptoms or a disease; not so used by physicians.

CONFABULATION — lying to conceal a faulty memory.

CONTUSION — bruising injury of any body tissue including the brain, spinal cord, or a nerve.

CONUS — the cone-shaped end of the spinal cord at about the level of the lowermost or twelfth rib.

CONVOLUTION — irregular protuberant part of the brain's surface; also called a gyrus.

*CONVULSION — sudden attack of violent uncontrollable muscle shaking, usually accompanied by loss of consciousness, such as may be caused by epilepsy or some drastic disturbance of brain circulation or chemistry.

'CORD, SPINAL — a continuation of the brainstem, protected by the SPINAL CANAL, which gives rise to NERVE ROOTS that unite outside the spine to form the nerves of the body.

CORDOTOMY — cutting of a small part of the spinal cord by surgery or by radio-frequency probe.

CORNEA — sensitive covering of the lens of the eye.

CORTISONE — synthetic preparation resembling a hormone formed by the outer layer or cortex of the ADRENAL GLANDS.

CRANIOPLASTY — cranial plastic surgery to repair a defect in the skull.

CRANIOTOMY — a surgical opening of the skull.

*CRANIUM (*adj.*, CRANIAL) — the skull.

CRYOTHERAPY — cold treatment, as by a highly cooled probe, for certain kinds of surgical procedures.

CYST — encapsulated cavity, usually round, containing fluid.

DEBRIDEMENT	thorough cleansing of a wound by trimming jagged edges of tissue and flushing with saline solution.
' DECOMPRESSION	surgical relief of pressure on the brain, spinal cord, or a spinal nerve root.
DEGENERATION OF A NERVE	withering of nerve fibers beyond the point of a serious nerve injury.
DENDRITE	one of the many fine short whiskerlike extensions of a nerve cell that connect it with other nerve cells and sometimes with nerve fibers.
DÉJÀ VU	French: a feeling that something has "already been seen" (or experienced), as in an aura preceding some epileptic attacks.
DISC	round cushion of cartilage between the bones of the spine.
DISLOCATION	slippage of one bone of a joint so that the bone is out of position.
DURA	the bluish, tough, protective membrane that lines the skull and bony canal of the spine.
DYSRHYTHMIA	disturbed rhythm, as in the "brain waves" during an epileptic attack.
DYSTONIA	a varying, severe disturbance of MUSCULAR TONE that leads to bizarre postures and posturing.
DYSTROPHY	disturbance of muscle size (literally, growth) that may make some muscles grossly enlarged and others too small.

ECHO TEST, ECHO-ENCEPHALOGRAM	test in which ultrasonic waves are passed from one side of the head to the other; their "echo" can indicate any shift or enlargement of the brain's ventricles and can detect some kinds of blood clot or brain tumor.
EDEMA	accumulation of fluid that can lead to congestion or swelling of body tissue.
ELECTROENCEPH-ALOGRAM (EEG)	graphic tracing of the electrical activity of the brain, which indicates any variations of rate, rhythm, and amplitude.
ELECTROMYOGRAM (EMG)	graphic tracing of the electrical activity of a muscle.
ELECTROSHOCK THERAPY (EST)	treatment of certain kinds of mental illness by passing an electric current through the head. Because it also causes a convulsion, it is sometimes described as electroconvulsive therapy (ECT). Not a neurosurgical procedure.
EMBOLISM (EM-BOLUS, *pl.* EM-BOLI)	any obstruction, such as a blood clot, fragment of tumor, or substance purposely introduced for treatment, that is carried along by the blood and may plug a blood vessel.
ENDOCRINE GLAND	gland of internal secretion, one which secretes or delivers its products (HOR-MONES) directly into the blood stream to be carried to other parts of the body. The adrenal, pineal, pituitary, thyroid, and sex glands are examples.

FASICULATION   rippling or twitching of muscles
                      caused by certain spinal cord or nerve
                      ailments, or sometimes by muscle fa-
                      tigue.

FONTANELLE   one of the apertures that exist in a
                      baby's skull before the skull bones
                      grow solidly together.

⁕ FRACTURE   break, as in a bone. Fractures may be
                      linear—a crack like a line; depressed
                      —pushed inward; compound—asso-
                      ciated with a break in the skin; or
                      comminuted—associated with several
                      fragments of damaged bone.

GANGLION (*pl.*,   group of nerve cells; *see* BASAL GANG-
GANGLIA)   LIA.

GLIA (*adj.*, GLIAL) supporting cells of the brain and
                      spinal cord, interspersed among their
                      nerve cells and nerve fibers.

GLIOMA   tumor composed of glial cells.

⁕ GRAY MATTER   portions of the brain and spinal cord
                      that look gray because of many
                      densely packed nerve cells; see also
                      WHITE MATTER.

GYRUS   see CONVOLUTION.

\ HEMATOMA   blood clot from a hemorrhage; may be
                      extradural—just outside the dural lin-
                      ing of the skull; subdural—just under
                      the dura; or intracerebral—inside the
                      substance of the brain.

HEMICRANIA   headache over one side of the head.

HEMISPHERECTOMY   surgical removal of one cerebral hemisphere, as for certain kinds of cerebral palsy.

HORMONE   a product of an ENDOCRINE GLAND; an example is adrenaline.

HYDROCEPHALUS   literally, "water on the brain"; excess of CEREBROSPINAL FLUID inside the skull, causing the ventricles of the brain to become distended.

HYPERTONIA   excessive MUSCULAR TONE, making muscles tense and muscle reflexes overactive.

HYPOPHYSIS   see PITUITARY GLAND.

HYPOPHYSECTOMY   operation to cut out the hypophysis or pituitary gland.

HYPOTONIA   unusually poor MUSCULAR TONE, usually because too few of the usual nerve signals reach the muscles.

LAMINA   the part of a VERTEBRA that forms an arch over the spinal cord.

LAMINECTOMY   cutting away all or part of a lamina.

LESION   medical term for anything that has physically interfered with any part of the body.

LIGATION   tying something, such as a blood vessel, with a thread or "suture."

LOBE   a rounded subdivision of a structure of the body, such as the frontal, parietal, occipital, and temporal lobes of the brain.

LOBOTOMY	cutting into or otherwise interrupting connections of a lobe of the brain.
' LUMBAR	the lower part of the spine, between the twelfth rib and the SACRUM.
LUMBAR PUNCTURE	see SPINAL TAP.
' MEDULLA	the lowermost and farthest-back portion of the BRAINSTEM where it merges with the spinal cord.
MENINGES (*adj.*, MENINGEAL)	the DURA and ARACHNOID membranes surrounding the brain and spinal cord.
MENINGIOMA	benign tumor arising from the meninges.
' MENINGITIS	inflammation of the meninges, usually from infection of the cerebrospinal fluid.
MENINGOMYEL-OCELE	faulty development of the meningeal membranes causing formation of a cyst filled with cerebrospinal fluid.
' METABOLISM	the chemical changes which take place in the process of living and growing.
METASTATIS (*adj.*, METASTATIC)	migration of disease from an original site to some other part of the body.
MICRONEURO-SURGERY	neurosurgery performed while the surgeon is looking through a binocular microscope.
MUSCULAR TONE	the degree of tautness or tension in a muscle that prevents it from being utterly relaxed and flabby. See HYPER-TONIA; HYPOTONIA; ATONIA.
MYELOGRAM	x-ray test for the detection of a slipped

	disc, tumor, etc., affecting the spinal cord or its nerve roots.
MYOPATHY	disease of muscle.
NEOPLASM	literally, new growth—a tumor.
NERVE	a short or long round flexible structure composed of nerve fibers enveloped by a covering called the nerve sheath.
NERVE BLOCK	process of "blocking" or deadening a nerve with a substance like Novocain or with alcohol for relief of pain or certain severe muscle spasms.
NERVE CELL (NEURON)	any cell in the body which gives rise to a nerve fiber and is capable of initiating or transmitting nerve signals.
NERVE, CRANIAL	a nerve of the brain itself. There are twelve on each side.
NERVE FIBER (AXON)	principal filamentous extension of a nerve; nerve fibers transmit the most important signals from a nerve cell, comprise the bulk of the WHITE MATTER of the brain and spinal cord, and are the "wires" of all nerves.
NERVE PATHWAY	compact bundle of nerve fibers within the brain or spinal cord.
PERIPHERAL NERVE	a nerve of the body.
NERVE REGENERA- TION	regrowth of nerve fibers along a damaged or surgically repaired nerve.
NERVE ROOT	small groups of nerve filaments within the spinal canal, which connect the nerves of the body with the spinal cord.

NERVE SHEATH   the covering of a nerve.

NERVOUS SYSTEM   the brain, spinal cord, and nerves of
                      the body.

NEURAL   pertaining to nerves or the nervous
                      system.

NEURALGIA   nerve pain.

NEURECTOMY   removal of part of a nerve.

NEURINOMA   benign tumor of a nerve.

NEURITIS   inflammation of a nerve.

NEUROLOGIST   specialist in the diagnosis and non-
                      surgical treatment of diseases and dis-
                      orders of the nervous system.

NEUROMA   lump of scar tissue in or around an
                      injured nerve.

NEURON   see NERVE CELL.

NEUROPATHY   disease of a nerve or nerves.

NEUROSURGEON   specialist in the surgical treatment of
                      disorders of the nervous system.

NEUROTRANS-   chemical substance essential for the
   MITTER   transmission of nerve signals across a
                      SYNAPSE.

NUCLEUS   (1) a small unit inside a cell, which
   (pl., NUCLEI)   controls the activity of the cell; (2) a
                      cluster of nerve cells within the brain.

OPHTHALMOSCOPE   instrument for inspecting the blood
                      vessels inside the eyeball and the op-
                      tic nerve.

OPTIC NERVE   nerve of vision.

PALSY	PARALYSIS.
PALSY, BELL'S	paralysis of the muscles on one side of the face.
PALSY, SHAKING	see PARKINSON'S DISEASE.
PARALYSIS	complete loss of voluntary control of a muscle.
PARESIS	weakness of a muscle or muscles: monoparesis—muscle weakness of one limb; paraparesis—muscle weakness of both legs; hemiparesis—muscle weakness on one side of the body.
PARKINSON'S DISEASE	rhythmic shaking of a limb or limbs, caused by disturbance of certain nerve cells in the brain.
PERNICIOUS ANEMIA (PA)	form of anemia that sometimes affects the spinal cord.
PHANTOM LIMB	sensation that an amputated limb is still present.
PHOTOPHOBIA	sensitivity to or fear of bright lights.
PINEAL GLAND	small gland of uncertain function, near the center of the brain.
PITUITARY GLAND	the so-called master gland, located in the SELLA TURCICA; its hormones regulate other ENDOCRINE GLANDS.
-PLEGIA	suffix indicating a form of PARALYSIS: monoplegia—of one limb; paraplegia—of both legs; quadraplegia—of all four limbs; hemiplegia—of one side of the body.

GLOSSARY

PNEUMOENCEPH-ALOGRAM (PEG) x-ray test which involves the introduction of air by a spinal tap to outline the brain.

POLIOMYELITIS virus infection of the spinal cord that can lead to temporary or permanent muscle paralysis and wasting.

POLYNEURITIS inflammation of several nerves.

PSYCHOMOTOR SEIZURE convulsion characterized by psychic or emotional disturbances as well as by muscle motor movements.

RHIZOTOMY cutting a nerve root for relief of pain or severe muscle spasm.

SACRUM the lower part of the spine between the last movable VERTEBRA and the COCCYX.

SCAN, RADIOACTIVE test for the detection of brain tumors and other disorders, including aberrations in the flow of the cerebrospinal fluid.

SELLA TURCICA tiny bone cavity, situated under the brain just back of the eyes and containing the PITUITARY GLAND.

SENSORY CELL nerve cell concerned with the detection or transmission of sensation.

SENSORY TRACT pathway of sensory nerve fibers in the brain or spinal cord; see SPINOTHALAMIC TRACT.

SHUNT a by-passing or shunting of fluid, such as cerebrospinal fluid or blood, around a point of obstruction.

SPASM   constriction, as of muscles or blood vessels.

SPASMODIC TORTI-
    COLLIS
    intermittent twitching of neck muscles such that the head is pulled downward and to one side.

SPINAL CANAL   flexible tube of bone which contains the spinal cord and its nerve branches called nerve roots.

SPINAL CORD   see CORD, SPINAL.

SPINAL FUSION   solid uniting of two bones by means of a bone graft; spontaneous fusion may occur as the result of injury, disease, or age.

SPINAL PROCESS   individual spikelike backward extension of a VERTEBRA that is one of the bony bumps one can see and feel along the length of one's spine.

SPINAL TAP   insertion of a needle, usually in the lower part of the spine below the level of the spinal cord, for analysis of cerebrospinal fluid.

SPINAL COLUMN   the spine; the column of spinal bones called VERTEBRAE; also known as the VERTEBRAL COLUMN.

SPINOTHALAMIC
    TRACT
    the bundle of sensory fibers in the spinal cord which run from the spine to the THALAMUS and are concerned with sensations of pain and temperature.

STEREOTAXIC PRO-
    CEDURE
    placement of a probe or similar small instrument in the brain or spinal cord,

under x-ray guidance, for purposes of treatment.

STROKE   sudden onset of symptoms of serious brain disturbance caused by localized impairment of the blood supply or by a hemorrhage; see also CEREBROVASCULAR ACCIDENT.

STUPOR   profound state of lethargy and mental blunting that is similar to but not as severe as COMA.

SYNAPSE   infinitesimally small gap which a nerve signal must cross; see NEUROTRANSMITTER.

THALAMUS   portion of the deep GRAY MATTER of the brain close to the BASAL GANGLIA.

THALAMOTOMY   surgical or stereotaxic interruption of a specific part of the thalamus for treatment of specific symptoms; for example, to relieve pain, intense anxiety, or certain kinds of otherwise incurable tremor.

THERMOGRAM   test to record temperature, such as that of the skin, by means of infrared rays.

THROMBOSIS (THROMBUS)   internal clotting of an artery or vein so that the flow of blood in that vessel is either reduced or completely blocked.

THYROID   endocrine gland in the front of the neck essential for normal body METABOLISM.

TIC DOULOUREUX — sudden intermittent acutely severe pains in the face along one or more of the three branches or divisions of the TRIGEMINAL NERVE.

TIC, MUSCULAR — an intermittent painless twitching of one or more muscles.

TRACHEA — the windpipe.

TRACHEOTOMY — cutting a small opening in the windpipe and inserting a plastic tube into it, for artificial respiration or suctioning of mucus.

TRIGEMINAL NERVE — the fifth cranial nerve, one on each side, for sensation of that side of the face and mouth and for chewing on that side.

TRIGEMINAL NEURALGIA, TRIGEMINAL TIC — other names for TIC DOULOUREUX.

VENTRICLE — small anatomical cavity; in the brain one of the four natural cavities filled with CEREBROSPINAL FLUID.

VENTRICULOGRAM — test whereby air or some other substance that shows up on x-rays is inserted directly into a ventricle of the brain for diagnostic purposes.

VERTEBRA (*pl.* VERTEBRAE) — bone of the spinal or vertebral column.

WHITE MATTER — the part of the brain and spinal cord which has a whitish color because it is composed mostly of NERVE FIBERS; see also GRAY MATTER.

For Further Reading

Cajal, Santiago Ramón y. *Recollections of My Life*. Translated from the third Spanish edition (1923) by E. Horne Craigie and Juan Cano. Cambridge, Mass.: M. I. T. Press, 1966.

Delgado, José M. R. *Physical Control of the Mind: Toward a Psychocivilized Society*. Edited by R. N. Anshen. New York: Harper & Row, 1969.

Dimond, E. Grey. "Acupuncture Anesthesia," *Journal of the American Medical Association*, December 6, 1971, pp. 1558–1563.

Downey, John A., and Darling, Robert C., eds. *Physiological Basis of Rehabilitation Medicine*. Philadelphia: W. B. Saunders Company, 1971.

Elliott, H. Chandler. *The Shape of Intelligence: The Evolution of the Human Brain*. New York: Charles Scribner's Sons, 1969.

Friedman, Arnold P., and Merritt, H. Houston, eds. *Head-*

ache: Diagnosis and Treatment. Philadelphia: F. A. Davis, 1959.

Fulton, John F. *Harvey Cushing: A Biography*. Springfield, Ill.: Charles C. Thomas, 1946.

Kinnier-Wilson, S. A. *Neurology*. 2 vols. Baltimore: Williams & Wilkins, 1940.

Kraus, Hans. *The Cause, Prevention and Treatment of Backache, Stress and Tension*. New York: Simon & Schuster, 1965.

Lennox, William G. *Science and Seizures: New Light on Epilepsy and Migraine*. 2d ed. New York: Harper, 1946.

Lennox, William G., and Lennox, M. A. *Epilepsy and Related Disorders*. 2 vols. London: J. & A. Churchill, 1960.

Livingston, Samuel, and Pruce, Irving M. *Living with Epileptic Seizures*. Springfield, Ill.: Charles C. Thomas, 1963.

Penfield, Wilder, and Jasper, Herbert. *Epilepsy and the Functional Anatomy of the Human Brain*. Boston: Little, Brown, 1954.

Pfeiffer, John. *The Human Brain*. New York: Harper, 1955.

Pool, J. Lawrence, and Potts, D. Gordon. *Aneurysms and Arteriovenous Malformations of the Brain*. New York: Harper & Row, 1965.

Willis, Thomas. *The Anatomy of the Brain and Nerves*. Edited by William Feindel. Tercentenary ed. 2 vols. Montreal: McGill University Press, 1965.

Wooldridge, Jean E. *The Machinery of the Brain*. New York: McGraw-Hill Book Company, 1963.

Index

J. Lawrence Pool, M.D. received his A.B. from Harvard in 1928 and his M.D. from Columbia in 1932. Dr. Pool practiced neurosurgery at Bellevue and other hospitals in and around New York City and also engaged in research leading to the degree of Doctor of Medical Science, Columbia University, in 1940. He was appointed to the staff of the Neurological Institute of Columbia-Presbyterian Medical Center, New York City, where he served for twenty-three years as Professor and Chairman of Neurological Surgery. He is now Emeritus Professor. Dr. Pool is the author of over 100 medical articles and author or co-author of four medical books.